LOW FODMAP JOURNAL

SPECIFICALLY DESIGNED FOR IRRITABLE BOWEL SYNDROME (IBS) PATIENTS

MONET MANBACCI, PH.D.

(Edition-1)

Copyright © 2020 Monet Manbacci

All Right Reserved.

ISBN: 9781655158513

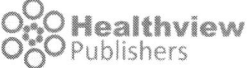

DISCLAIMER NOTICE

No part of this publication may be reproduced, distributed, or transmitted in any form or by any means, including photocopying, recording, or other electronic or mechanical methods, or by any information storage and retrieval system without the prior written permission of the publisher, except in the case of very brief quotations embodied in critical reviews and certain other noncommercial uses permitted by copyright law. Please, consider that the information in this journal is only for educational purposes. No warranties of any kind are implied or declared in this journal. Readers acknowledge that the author of this journal is not engaged in the rendering of medical, legal, financial, or professional advice. Hence, consult a licensed professional before applying any hints, tips, or techniques outlined in this journal. By reading this notice, the readers agree that the author of this journal is not responsible for any direct or indirect losses that are incurred because of the use of the information contained in this journal, including but not limited to inaccuracies, omissions, and errors.

Table of Contents

Preface 4
    How to Use this Journal 5
My Low FODMAP Journal 6
    Daily Records 6
    Biweekly Meal Plan-1 113
    Biweekly Meal Plan-2 114
    Low FODMAP Comprehensive Food List 115
Notes 123
Last Words 125
    About The Author 125
    Other Books By Monet Manbacci 125

Preface

If you or your loved one has been diagnosed with Inflammatory Bowel Syndrome (IBS), you already know how hard this syndrome could be and how tough the IBS can be managed. Rsearch studies have found that many of the IBS problems, come from the followings:
- Not knowing much about IBS
- Self-treatment
- Ignoring signs and symptoms
- Not following the doctor's orders correctly or completely
- Mismanagement of the disease

One of the best ways to manage your IBS, which **helps you manage your symptoms better, and have a healthier life**, is to follow Low FODMAP diet, with the help of a comprehensive Low FODMAP journal.

FODMAP stands for stands for **f**ermentable **o**ligo-, **d**i-, **m**ono-saccharides **a**nd **p**olyols. These are short-chain sugars that some research studies say that they can irritate the guts in people with IBS. Studies showed that having a Low FODMAP diet, which is simply to avoid or reduce consuming FODMAP sugars for a period of time (e.g., to months) and then re-introduce foods to the body might be effective in healing many IBS patients.

This journal provides you with **a practical and easy-to-use platform** to record your daily meals and IBS conditions. You can easily use your journal on a daily basis and record your trigerring foods, symptoms, fluid intake, stress level, bowel movement, and other info you may want to recall. The platform designed for daily records is simple and easy to use. You can record necessary information mostly by check-marking and by writing a few words. Remember that it is extremely valuable to put only 2-3 minutes every day to **proactively track your health and manage your IBS**. Each week, you can summarize your diet adherence and IBS conditions as well. This journal provides you with three months of daily records, comprehensive lists of foods to avoid and foods to consume based on Low FODMAP diet, and two blank pages to record your bi-weekly meal plans for your IBS.

How to Use this Journal

Using this Low FODMAP journal is very simple. You just need to answer yes/no questions by check-marking, and add any notes you wish by writing few words.

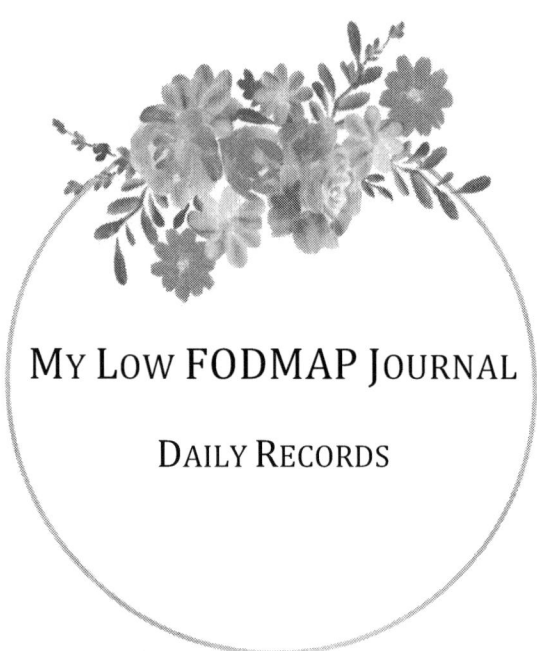

My Low FODMAP Journal

Daily Records

Date: _____   Mon Tue Wed Thu Fri Sat Sun

Quote of the Day:
"Life is not a problem. To look at it as a problem is to take a wrong step. It is a mystery to be lived, loved, and experienced." - Osho

Your Mood Today

Stress Level:
0 1 2 3 4 5 6 7 8 9 10
No Stress — Full Stress

Sleep Quality:
0 1 2 3 4 5 6 7 8 9 10
Very bad — Very well

How long did you sleep last night? _____ Hrs.

Time	Meals Taken Today	Symptoms Experienced:	How intense? (1: low, 5: severe)
	Breakfast:		
	Lunch:		
	Dinner:		
	Snacks:		

Bowel Movement:
How many liquid bowel movements you had today?

One:	Two:	Three:	Four:	More than 4:

Did you have any of the followings today?

Bowel Urgency: YES NO
Bleeding: YES NO
Partial evacuation: YES NO
Sinking defecation: YES NO

Mucus in the stool: YES NO
Painful bowel movement: YES NO
High pressure evacuation: YES NO
Other Symptoms: YES NO

Stool Type:

1. Very constipated: YES NO
2. Constipated: YES NO
3. Normal sausage-like: YES NO
4. Normal smooth: YES NO
5. Soft blobs: YES NO
6. Mushy: YES NO
7. Liquid: YES NO
Any Notes:

Activities:
Did you have a workout today? YES NO
Was it intense? YES NO
Your weight changed today? YES NO
How many glasses of water did you have? _____

How long did you have workout? _____ Min.
Did you have a good appetite? YES NO
Did you have time to meditate or practice Yoga today? YES NO

Date: _____   Mon Tue Wed Thu Fri Sat Sun
                  ○   ○   ○   ○   ○   ○   ○

Quote of the Day:
"Let the beauty of what you love, be what you do."
- Rumi

Your Mood Today [ ][ ][ ][ ][ ][ ]

Stress Level:
0 1 2 3 4 5 6 7 8 9 10
No Stress   Full Stress

Sleep Quality:
0 1 2 3 4 5 6 7 8 9 10
Very bad   Very well

How long did you sleep last night? _____ Hrs.

Time	Meals Taken Today	Symptoms Experienced:	How intense? (1: low, 5: severe)
	Breakfast:		
	Lunch:		
	Dinner:		
	Snacks:		

Bowel Movement:
How many liquid bowel movements you had today?

| One: | Two: | Three: | Four: | More than 4: |

Did you have any of the followings today?

Bowel Urgency: YES NO
Bleeding: YES NO
Partial evacuation: YES NO
Sinking defecation: YES NO

Mucus in the stool: YES NO
Painful bowel movement: YES NO
High pressure evacuation: YES NO
Other Symptoms: YES NO

Stool Type:

1. Very constipated: YES NO
2. Constipated: YES NO
3. Normal sausage-like: YES NO
4. Normal smooth: YES NO
5. Soft blobs: YES NO
6. Mushy: YES NO
7. Liquid: YES NO
Any Notes:

Activities:

Did you have a workout today? YES NO
Was it intense? YES NO
How long did you have workout? ____ Min.
Your weight changed today? YES NO
Did you have a good appetite? YES NO
How many glasses of water did you have? ____
Did you have time to meditate or practice Yoga today? YES NO

Date: _____   Mon Tue Wed Thu Fri Sat Sun

Quote of the Day:
> "Learn this from water: loud splashes the brook, but the depth of the ocean is calm."
> - Buddha

Your Mood Today

Stress Level: 0 — 10 (No Stress — Full Stress)

Sleep Quality: 0 — 10 (Very bad — Very well)

How long did you sleep last night? _____ Hrs.

Time	Meals Taken Today	Symptoms Experienced:	How intense? (1: low, 5: severe)
	Breakfast:		
	Lunch:		
	Dinner:		
	Snacks:		

Bowel Movement:

How many liquid bowel movements you had today?
| One: | Two: | Three: | Four: | More than 4: |

Did you have any of the followings today?

Bowel Urgency: YES NO
Bleeding: YES NO
Partial evacuation: YES NO
Sinking defecation: YES NO

Mucus in the stool: YES NO
Painful bowel movement: YES NO
High pressure evacuation: YES NO
Other Symptoms: YES NO

Stool Type:

1. Very constipated: YES NO
2. Constipated: YES NO
3. Normal sausage-like: YES NO
4. Normal smooth: YES NO
5. Soft blobs: YES NO
6. Mushy: YES NO
7. Liquid: YES NO
Any Notes:

Activities:

Did you have a workout today? YES NO
Was it intense? YES NO
Your weight changed today? YES NO
How many glasses of water did you have? _____

How long did you have workout? ____ Min.
Did you have a good appetite? YES NO
Did you have time to meditate or practice Yoga today? YES NO

Date: _____   Mon Tue Wed Thu Fri Sat Sun
○ ○ ○ ○ ○ ○ ○

Quote of the Day:
> "Turn yourself not away from three best things: Good Thought, Good Word, and Good Deed." - Zoroaster

Your Mood Today [ ][ ][ ][ ][ ]

Stress Level:
0 1 2 3 4 5 6 7 8 9 10
No Stress — Full Stress

Sleep Quality:
0 1 2 3 4 5 6 7 8 9 10
Very bad — Very well

How long did you sleep last night? _____ Hrs.

Time	Meals Taken Today	Symptoms Experienced:	How intense? (1: low, 5: severe)
	Breakfast:		
	Lunch:		
	Dinner:		
	Snacks:		

Bowel Movement:
How many liquid bowel movements you had today?
| One: | Two: | Three: | Four: | More than 4: |

Did you have any of the followings today?

Bowel Urgency: YES NO
Bleeding: YES NO
Partial evacuation: YES NO
Sinking defecation: YES NO
Mucus in the stool: YES NO
Painful bowel movement: YES NO
High pressure evacuation: YES NO
Other Symptoms: YES NO

Stool Type:

1. Very constipated: YES NO
2. Constipated: YES NO
3. Normal sausage-like: YES NO
4. Normal smooth: YES NO
5. Soft blobs: YES NO
6. Mushy: YES NO
7. Liquid: YES NO
Any Notes:

Activities:

Did you have a workout today? YES NO
Was it intense? YES NO
How long did you have workout? ____ Min.
Your weight changed today? YES NO
Did you have a good appetite? YES NO
How many glasses of water did you have? _____
Did you have time to meditate or practice Yoga today? YES NO

Date: _____   Mon Tue Wed Thu Fri Sat Sun
                  ○   ○   ○   ○   ○   ○   ○

Quote of the Day:

> "When I let go of what I am, I become what I might be."
> - Lao Tzu

Your Mood Today [ ] [ ] [ ] [ ] [ ] [ ]

Stress Level: 0 1 2 3 4 5 6 7 8 9 10
No Stress   Full Stress

Sleep Quality: 0 1 2 3 4 5 6 7 8 9 10
Very bad   Very well

How long did you sleep last night? _____ Hrs.

Time	Meals Taken Today	Symptoms Experienced:	How intense? (1: low, 5: severe)
	Breakfast:		
	Lunch:		
	Dinner:		
	Snacks:		

Bowel Movement:

How many liquid bowel movements you had today?

| One: | Two: | Three: | Four: | More than 4: |

Did you have any of the followings today?

Bowel Urgency: YES NO
Bleeding: YES NO
Partial evacuation: YES NO
Sinking defecation: YES NO

Mucus in the stool: YES NO
Painful bowel movement: YES NO
High pressure evacuation: YES NO
Other Symptoms: YES NO

Stool Type:

1. Very constipated: YES NO
2. Constipated: YES NO
3. Normal sausage-like: YES NO
4. Normal smooth: YES NO
5. Soft blobs: YES NO
6. Mushy: YES NO
7. Liquid: YES NO
Any Notes:

Activities:

Did you have a workout today? YES NO
Was it intense? YES NO
How long did you have workout? ____ Min.
Your weight changed today? YES NO
Did you have a good appetite? YES NO
How many glasses of water did you have? ____
Did you have time to meditate or practice Yoga today? YES NO

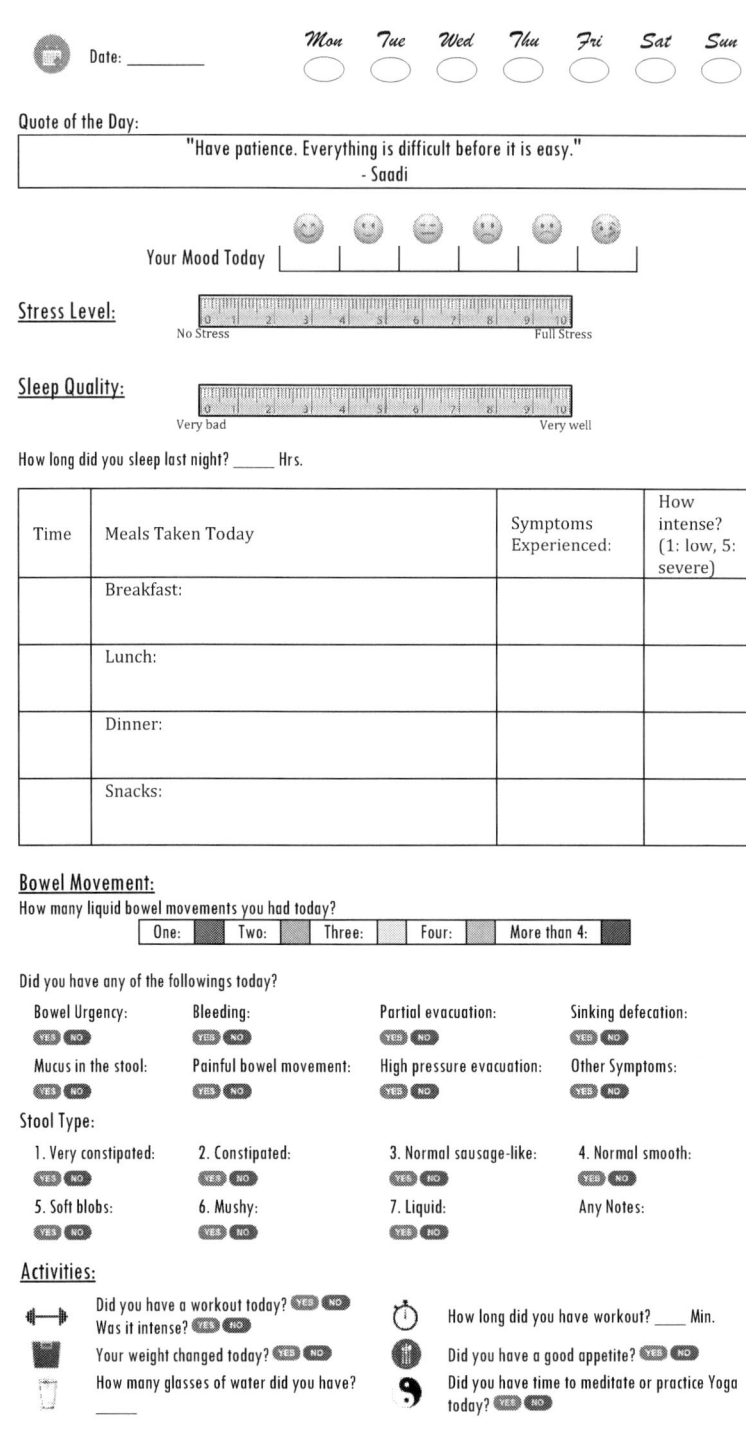

Date: _____ Mon Tue Wed Thu Fri Sat Sun

Quote of the Day:
> "You can only be afraid of what you think you know."
> - Jiddu Krishnamurti

Your Mood Today [ ] [ ] [ ] [ ] [ ] [ ]

Stress Level:
0 — 10 (No Stress — Full Stress)

Sleep Quality:
0 — 10 (Very bad — Very well)

How long did you sleep last night? _____ Hrs.

Time	Meals Taken Today	Symptoms Experienced:	How intense? (1: low, 5: severe)
	Breakfast:		
	Lunch:		
	Dinner:		
	Snacks:		

Bowel Movement:
How many liquid bowel movements you had today?

| One: | Two: | Three: | Four: | More than 4: |

Did you have any of the followings today?

Bowel Urgency: YES NO
Bleeding: YES NO
Partial evacuation: YES NO
Sinking defecation: YES NO

Mucus in the stool: YES NO
Painful bowel movement: YES NO
High pressure evacuation: YES NO
Other Symptoms: YES NO

Stool Type:

1. Very constipated: YES NO
2. Constipated: YES NO
3. Normal sausage-like: YES NO
4. Normal smooth: YES NO

5. Soft blobs: YES NO
6. Mushy: YES NO
7. Liquid: YES NO
Any Notes:

Activities:

Did you have a workout today? YES NO
Was it intense? YES NO

How long did you have workout? ____ Min.

Your weight changed today? YES NO

Did you have a good appetite? YES NO

How many glasses of water did you have? _____

Did you have time to meditate or practice Yoga today? YES NO

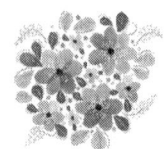

Week-1 IBS Control Record

Did you miss any activity due to your IBS condition?	YES NO
Do you think your IBS controlled well last week?	YES NO
Were you happy with your current treatment last week?	YES NO
Did you feel pain or discomfort last week?	YES NO
Did you have a good eating appetite last week?	YES NO
Did you feel fatigued last week?	YES NO
Did you feel depressed/anxious last week due to your IBS?	YES NO
Do you think you lost weight last week?	YES NO
Do you feel your bowel symptoms got better last week?	YES NO

Low FODMAP Diet Adherence:

Did you have any of the following foods this week?

Alcohol: YES NO	Chocolate: YES NO	Coffee: YES NO
Soda: YES NO	Sweet Fruits: YES NO	Lactose Products: YES NO
Fatty/greasy Foods: YES NO	Fried Foods: YES NO	Gluten Products: YES NO
FODMAP Sugars: YES NO	Raw Vegetables: YES NO	Spicy Foods: YES NO

Add any other suspicious foods you consumed: Did you get any discomfort?

1. _____ YES NO
2. _____ YES NO
3. _____ YES NO
4. _____ YES NO
5. _____ YES NO
6. _____ YES NO
7. _____ YES NO
8. _____ YES NO
9. _____ YES NO
10. _____ YES NO

Others:

Medications/Supplements taken this week: _____

Tell a good thing that happened this week: _____

Other Notes: _____
_____
_____
_____
_____

Date: _____   Mon Tue Wed Thu Fri Sat Sun

Quote of the Day:

"Between me and you, there is only me. Take away the "Me," so only you remain."
- Mansur Hallaj

Your Mood Today

Stress Level:
0 1 2 3 4 5 6 7 8 9 10
No Stress   Full Stress

Sleep Quality:
0 1 2 3 4 5 6 7 8 9 10
Very bad   Very well

How long did you sleep last night? _____ Hrs.

Time	Meals Taken Today	Symptoms Experienced:	How intense? (1: low, 5: severe)
	Breakfast:		
	Lunch:		
	Dinner:		
	Snacks:		

Bowel Movement:

How many liquid bowel movements you had today?

| One: | Two: | Three: | Four: | More than 4: |

Did you have any of the followings today?

Bowel Urgency: YES NO
Bleeding: YES NO
Partial evacuation: YES NO
Sinking defecation: YES NO

Mucus in the stool: YES NO
Painful bowel movement: YES NO
High pressure evacuation: YES NO
Other Symptoms: YES NO

Stool Type:

1. Very constipated: YES NO
2. Constipated: YES NO
3. Normal sausage-like: YES NO
4. Normal smooth: YES NO
5. Soft blobs: YES NO
6. Mushy: YES NO
7. Liquid: YES NO
Any Notes:

Activities:

Did you have a workout today? YES NO
Was it intense? YES NO
Your weight changed today? YES NO
How many glasses of water did you have? _____

How long did you have workout? ____ Min.
Did you have a good appetite? YES NO
Did you have time to meditate or practice Yoga today? YES NO

Date: _____   Mon Tue Wed Thu Fri Sat Sun
                    ○   ○   ○   ○   ○   ○   ○

Quote of the Day:

> "Love is the goal; life is the journey."
> - Osho

Your Mood Today ☺ 🙂 😐 🙁 ☹

Stress Level:
0 1 2 3 4 5 6 7 8 9 10
No Stress   Full Stress

Sleep Quality:
0 1 2 3 4 5 6 7 8 9 10
Very bad   Very well

How long did you sleep last night? _____ Hrs.

Time	Meals Taken Today	Symptoms Experienced:	How intense? (1: low, 5: severe)
	Breakfast:		
	Lunch:		
	Dinner:		
	Snacks:		

Bowel Movement:

How many liquid bowel movements you had today?

| One: | Two: | Three: | Four: | More than 4: |

Did you have any of the followings today?

Bowel Urgency: Bleeding: Partial evacuation: Sinking defecation:
YES NO   YES NO   YES NO   YES NO

Mucus in the stool: Painful bowel movement: High pressure evacuation: Other Symptoms:
YES NO   YES NO   YES NO   YES NO

Stool Type:

1. Very constipated: 2. Constipated: 3. Normal sausage-like: 4. Normal smooth:
YES NO   YES NO   YES NO   YES NO

5. Soft blobs: 6. Mushy: 7. Liquid: Any Notes:
YES NO   YES NO   YES NO

Activities:

Did you have a workout today? YES NO   How long did you have workout? ____ Min.
Was it intense? YES NO

Your weight changed today? YES NO   Did you have a good appetite? YES NO

How many glasses of water did you have?   Did you have time to meditate or practice Yoga
_____   today? YES NO

Date: _____   Mon Tue Wed Thu Fri Sat Sun

Quote of the Day:

> "What hurts you, blesses you. Darkness is your candle."
> - Rumi

Your Mood Today

Stress Level: 0 1 2 3 4 5 6 7 8 9 10
No Stress   Full Stress

Sleep Quality: 0 1 2 3 4 5 6 7 8 9 10
Very bad   Very well

How long did you sleep last night? _____ Hrs.

Time	Meals Taken Today	Symptoms Experienced:	How intense? (1: low, 5: severe)
	Breakfast:		
	Lunch:		
	Dinner:		
	Snacks:		

Bowel Movement:

How many liquid bowel movements you had today?
One: ___ Two: ___ Three: ___ Four: ___ More than 4: ___

Did you have any of the followings today?

Bowel Urgency: YES NO
Bleeding: YES NO
Partial evacuation: YES NO
Sinking defecation: YES NO

Mucus in the stool: YES NO
Painful bowel movement: YES NO
High pressure evacuation: YES NO
Other Symptoms: YES NO

Stool Type:

1. Very constipated: YES NO
2. Constipated: YES NO
3. Normal sausage-like: YES NO
4. Normal smooth: YES NO
5. Soft blobs: YES NO
6. Mushy: YES NO
7. Liquid: YES NO
Any Notes:

Activities:

Did you have a workout today? YES NO
Was it intense? YES NO

How long did you have workout? ____ Min.

Your weight changed today? YES NO

Did you have a good appetite? YES NO

How many glasses of water did you have? _____

Did you have time to meditate or practice Yoga today? YES NO

Date: _____ ○ Mon ○ Tue ○ Wed ○ Thu ○ Fri ○ Sat ○ Sun

Quote of the Day:
> "I never see what has been done; I only see what remains to be done."
> - Buddha

Your Mood Today: [😊][🙂][😐][🙁][😟][😣]

Stress Level:
0 1 2 3 4 5 6 7 8 9 10
No Stress — Full Stress

Sleep Quality:
0 1 2 3 4 5 6 7 8 9 10
Very bad — Very well

How long did you sleep last night? _____ Hrs.

Time	Meals Taken Today	Symptoms Experienced:	How intense? (1: low, 5: severe)
	Breakfast:		
	Lunch:		
	Dinner:		
	Snacks:		

Bowel Movement:

How many liquid bowel movements you had today?
One: ▢   Two: ▢   Three: ▢   Four: ▢   More than 4: ▢

Did you have any of the followings today?

Bowel Urgency: YES NO
Bleeding: YES NO
Partial evacuation: YES NO
Sinking defecation: YES NO

Mucus in the stool: YES NO
Painful bowel movement: YES NO
High pressure evacuation: YES NO
Other Symptoms: YES NO

Stool Type:

1. Very constipated: YES NO
2. Constipated: YES NO
3. Normal sausage-like: YES NO
4. Normal smooth: YES NO

5. Soft blobs: YES NO
6. Mushy: YES NO
7. Liquid: YES NO
Any Notes:

Activities:

Did you have a workout today? YES NO
Was it intense? YES NO
How long did you have workout? _____ Min.
Your weight changed today? YES NO
Did you have a good appetite? YES NO
How many glasses of water did you have? _____
Did you have time to meditate or practice Yoga today? YES NO

Date: _____   Mon Tue Wed Thu Fri Sat Sun

Quote of the Day:

> "The truth is not always beautiful, nor beautiful words the truth."
> - Lao Tzu

Your Mood Today

Stress Level: 0 - 10 (No Stress — Full Stress)

Sleep Quality: 0 - 10 (Very bad — Very well)

How long did you sleep last night? _____ Hrs.

Time	Meals Taken Today	Symptoms Experienced:	How intense? (1: low, 5: severe)
	Breakfast:		
	Lunch:		
	Dinner:		
	Snacks:		

Bowel Movement:

How many liquid bowel movements you had today?

| One: | Two: | Three: | Four: | More than 4: |

Did you have any of the followings today?

- Bowel Urgency: YES NO
- Bleeding: YES NO
- Partial evacuation: YES NO
- Sinking defecation: YES NO
- Mucus in the stool: YES NO
- Painful bowel movement: YES NO
- High pressure evacuation: YES NO
- Other Symptoms: YES NO

Stool Type:

1. Very constipated: YES NO
2. Constipated: YES NO
3. Normal sausage-like: YES NO
4. Normal smooth: YES NO
5. Soft blobs: YES NO
6. Mushy: YES NO
7. Liquid: YES NO

Any Notes:

Activities:

- Did you have a workout today? YES NO
- Was it intense? YES NO
- How long did you have workout? ____ Min.
- Your weight changed today? YES NO
- Did you have a good appetite? YES NO
- How many glasses of water did you have? _____
- Did you have time to meditate or practice Yoga today? YES NO

Date: _____   Mon Tue Wed Thu Fri Sat Sun
                     ○   ○   ○   ○   ○   ○   ○

Quote of the Day:

> "Victory comes from finding opportunities in problems."
> - Sun Tzu

Your Mood Today [😊] [🙂] [😐] [🙁] [😞]

Stress Level:

0 1 2 3 4 5 6 7 8 9 10
No Stress   Full Stress

Sleep Quality:

0 1 2 3 4 5 6 7 8 9 10
Very bad   Very well

How long did you sleep last night? _____ Hrs.

Time	Meals Taken Today	Symptoms Experienced:	How intense? (1: low, 5: severe)
	Breakfast:		
	Lunch:		
	Dinner:		
	Snacks:		

Bowel Movement:

How many liquid bowel movements you had today?

| One: | Two: | Three: | Four: | More than 4: |

Did you have any of the followings today?

Bowel Urgency: Bleeding: Partial evacuation: Sinking defecation:
YES NO   YES NO   YES NO   YES NO

Mucus in the stool: Painful bowel movement: High pressure evacuation: Other Symptoms:
YES NO   YES NO   YES NO   YES NO

Stool Type:

1. Very constipated: 2. Constipated: 3. Normal sausage-like: 4. Normal smooth:
YES NO   YES NO   YES NO   YES NO

5. Soft blobs: 6. Mushy: 7. Liquid: Any Notes:
YES NO   YES NO   YES NO

Activities:

Did you have a workout today? YES NO   How long did you have workout? ____ Min.
Was it intense? YES NO
Your weight changed today? YES NO   Did you have a good appetite? YES NO
How many glasses of water did you have? Did you have time to meditate or practice Yoga
_____   today? YES NO

Date: _____   Mon Tue Wed Thu Fri Sat Sun

Quote of the Day:
"I live my life based on two principles. One, I live as if today was my last day on earth. Two, I live today as if I am going to live forever." - Osho

Your Mood Today | 😊 | 🙂 | 😐 | 🙁 | ☹️ | 😣 |

Stress Level: 0–10 (No Stress — Full Stress)

Sleep Quality: 0–10 (Very bad — Very well)

How long did you sleep last night? _____ Hrs.

Time	Meals Taken Today	Symptoms Experienced:	How intense? (1: low, 5: severe)
	Breakfast:		
	Lunch:		
	Dinner:		
	Snacks:		

Bowel Movement:

How many liquid bowel movements you had today?
| One: | Two: | Three: | Four: | More than 4: |

Did you have any of the followings today?

Bowel Urgency: YES NO
Bleeding: YES NO
Partial evacuation: YES NO
Sinking defecation: YES NO

Mucus in the stool: YES NO
Painful bowel movement: YES NO
High pressure evacuation: YES NO
Other Symptoms: YES NO

Stool Type:

1. Very constipated: YES NO
2. Constipated: YES NO
3. Normal sausage-like: YES NO
4. Normal smooth: YES NO
5. Soft blobs: YES NO
6. Mushy: YES NO
7. Liquid: YES NO
Any Notes:

Activities:

Did you have a workout today? YES NO
Was it intense? YES NO

How long did you have workout? _____ Min.

Your weight changed today? YES NO

Did you have a good appetite? YES NO

How many glasses of water did you have? _____

Did you have time to meditate or practice Yoga today? YES NO

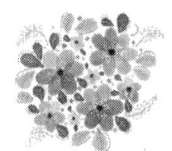

Week-2 IBS Control Record

Did you miss any activity due to your IBS condition?	YES NO
Do you think your IBS controlled well last week?	YES NO
Were you happy with your current treatment last week?	YES NO
Did you feel pain or discomfort last week?	YES NO
Did you have a good eating appetite last week?	YES NO
Did you feel fatigued last week?	YES NO
Did you feel depressed/anxious last week due to your IBS?	YES NO
Do you think you lost weight last week?	YES NO
Do you feel your bowel symptoms got better last week?	YES NO

Low FODMAP Diet Adherence:

Did you have any of the following foods this week?

FODMAP

Alcohol:	YES NO	Chocolate:	YES NO	Coffee:	YES NO
Soda:	YES NO	Sweet Fruits	YES NO	Lactose Products:	YES NO
Fatty/greasy Foods:	YES NO	Fried Foods:	YES NO	Gluten Products:	YES NO
FODMAP Sugars	YES NO	Raw Vegetables:	YES NO	Spicy Foods:	YES NO

Add any other suspicious foods you consumed: Did you get any discomfort?

1. _____ YES NO
2. _____ YES NO
3. _____ YES NO
4. _____ YES NO
5. _____ YES NO
6. _____ YES NO
7. _____ YES NO
8. _____ YES NO
9. _____ YES NO
10. _____ YES NO

Others:

Medications/Supplements taken this week: _____

Tell a good thing that happened this week: _____
_____

Other Notes:_____
_____
_____
_____
_____

Date: _____   Mon Tue Wed Thu Fri Sat Sun

Quote of the Day:
"We are shaped by our thoughts; we become what we think. When the mind is pure, joy follows like a shadow that never leaves." - Buddha

Your Mood Today | | | | | | |

<u>Stress Level:</u> 0 — 10   No Stress — Full Stress

<u>Sleep Quality:</u> 0 — 10   Very bad — Very well

How long did you sleep last night? _____ Hrs.

Time	Meals Taken Today	Symptoms Experienced:	How intense? (1: low, 5: severe)
	Breakfast:		
	Lunch:		
	Dinner:		
	Snacks:		

Bowel Movement:

How many liquid bowel movements you had today?
One: ▢ Two: ▢ Three: ▢ Four: ▢ More than 4: ▢

Did you have any of the followings today?

Bowel Urgency: YES NO
Bleeding: YES NO
Partial evacuation: YES NO
Sinking defecation: YES NO

Mucus in the stool: YES NO
Painful bowel movement: YES NO
High pressure evacuation: YES NO
Other Symptoms: YES NO

Stool Type:

1. Very constipated: YES NO
2. Constipated: YES NO
3. Normal sausage-like: YES NO
4. Normal smooth: YES NO

5. Soft blobs: YES NO
6. Mushy: YES NO
7. Liquid: YES NO
Any Notes:

Activities:

Did you have a workout today? YES NO
Was it intense? YES NO

How long did you have workout? _____ Min.

Your weight changed today? YES NO

Did you have a good appetite? YES NO

How many glasses of water did you have? _____

Did you have time to meditate or practice Yoga today? YES NO

Date: _____   Mon Tue Wed Thu Fri Sat Sun

Quote of the Day:

> "Success depends upon previous preparation, and without such preparation, there is sure to be a failure." - Confucius

Your Mood Today

Stress Level: 0 — 10 (No Stress — Full Stress)

Sleep Quality: 0 — 10 (Very bad — Very well)

How long did you sleep last night? _____ Hrs.

Time	Meals Taken Today	Symptoms Experienced:	How intense? (1: low, 5: severe)
	Breakfast:		
	Lunch:		
	Dinner:		
	Snacks:		

Bowel Movement:

How many liquid bowel movements you had today?

One: Two: Three: Four: More than 4:

Did you have any of the followings today?

Bowel Urgency: YES NO
Bleeding: YES NO
Partial evacuation: YES NO
Sinking defecation: YES NO

Mucus in the stool: YES NO
Painful bowel movement: YES NO
High pressure evacuation: YES NO
Other Symptoms: YES NO

Stool Type:

1. Very constipated: YES NO
2. Constipated: YES NO
3. Normal sausage-like: YES NO
4. Normal smooth: YES NO
5. Soft blobs: YES NO
6. Mushy: YES NO
7. Liquid: YES NO
Any Notes:

Activities:

Did you have a workout today? YES NO
Was it intense? YES NO

How long did you have workout? _____ Min.

Your weight changed today? YES NO

Did you have a good appetite? YES NO

How many glasses of water did you have? _____

Did you have time to meditate or practice Yoga today? YES NO

Date: _____ Mon Tue Wed Thu Fri Sat Sun

Quote of the Day:
> "Wherever you are is the entry point."
> - Kabir

Your Mood Today

Stress Level:
0 1 2 3 4 5 6 7 8 9 10
No Stress — Full Stress

Sleep Quality:
0 1 2 3 4 5 6 7 8 9 10
Very bad — Very well

How long did you sleep last night? _____ Hrs.

Time	Meals Taken Today	Symptoms Experienced:	How intense? (1: low, 5: severe)
	Breakfast:		
	Lunch:		
	Dinner:		
	Snacks:		

Bowel Movement:

How many liquid bowel movements you had today?
| One: | Two: | Three: | Four: | More than 4: |

Did you have any of the followings today?

Bowel Urgency: YES NO
Bleeding: YES NO
Partial evacuation: YES NO
Sinking defecation: YES NO

Mucus in the stool: YES NO
Painful bowel movement: YES NO
High pressure evacuation: YES NO
Other Symptoms: YES NO

Stool Type:

1. Very constipated: YES NO
2. Constipated: YES NO
3. Normal sausage-like: YES NO
4. Normal smooth: YES NO

5. Soft blobs: YES NO
6. Mushy: YES NO
7. Liquid: YES NO
Any Notes:

Activities:

Did you have a workout today? YES NO
Was it intense? YES NO
Your weight changed today? YES NO
How many glasses of water did you have? _____

How long did you have workout? ____ Min.
Did you have a good appetite? YES NO
Did you have time to meditate or practice Yoga today? YES NO

Date: _____ Mon ○ Tue ○ Wed ○ Thu ○ Fri ○ Sat ○ Sun ○

Quote of the Day:

"Every journey begins with a single step."
- Lao Tzu

Your Mood Today | | | | | |

Stress Level: 0–10 (No Stress — Full Stress)

Sleep Quality: 0–10 (Very bad — Very well)

How long did you sleep last night? _____ Hrs.

Time	Meals Taken Today	Symptoms Experienced:	How intense? (1: low, 5: severe)
	Breakfast:		
	Lunch:		
	Dinner:		
	Snacks:		

Bowel Movement:

How many liquid bowel movements you had today?

| One: | Two: | Three: | Four: | More than 4: |

Did you have any of the followings today?

Bowel Urgency: YES NO
Bleeding: YES NO
Partial evacuation: YES NO
Sinking defecation: YES NO

Mucus in the stool: YES NO
Painful bowel movement: YES NO
High pressure evacuation: YES NO
Other Symptoms: YES NO

Stool Type:

1. Very constipated: YES NO
2. Constipated: YES NO
3. Normal sausage-like: YES NO
4. Normal smooth: YES NO

5. Soft blobs: YES NO
6. Mushy: YES NO
7. Liquid: YES NO
Any Notes:

Activities:

Did you have a workout today? YES NO
Was it intense? YES NO
Your weight changed today? YES NO
How many glasses of water did you have? _____

How long did you have workout? _____ Min.
Did you have a good appetite? YES NO
Did you have time to meditate or practice Yoga today? YES NO

Date: _____   *Mon* ○ *Tue* ○ *Wed* ○ *Thu* ○ *Fri* ○ *Sat* ○ *Sun* ○

Quote of the Day:
> "You are not a drop in the ocean. You are the entire ocean in a drop."
> - Rumi

Your Mood Today: [😊] [🙂] [😐] [🙁] [☹] [😣]

Stress Level:
0 — 1 — 2 — 3 — 4 — 5 — 6 — 7 — 8 — 9 — 10
No Stress   Full Stress

Sleep Quality:
0 — 1 — 2 — 3 — 4 — 5 — 6 — 7 — 8 — 9 — 10
Very bad   Very well

How long did you sleep last night? _____ Hrs.

Time	Meals Taken Today	Symptoms Experienced:	How intense? (1: low, 5: severe)
	Breakfast:		
	Lunch:		
	Dinner:		
	Snacks:		

Bowel Movement:
How many liquid bowel movements you had today?

One:	Two:	Three:	Four:	More than 4:

Did you have any of the followings today?

Bowel Urgency: YES NO
Bleeding: YES NO
Partial evacuation: YES NO
Sinking defecation: YES NO

Mucus in the stool: YES NO
Painful bowel movement: YES NO
High pressure evacuation: YES NO
Other Symptoms: YES NO

Stool Type:

1. Very constipated: YES NO
2. Constipated: YES NO
3. Normal sausage-like: YES NO
4. Normal smooth: YES NO
5. Soft blobs: YES NO
6. Mushy: YES NO
7. Liquid: YES NO
Any Notes:

Activities:

Did you have a workout today? YES NO
Was it intense? YES NO

How long did you have workout? ____ Min.

Your weight changed today? YES NO

Did you have a good appetite? YES NO

How many glasses of water did you have? _____

Did you have time to meditate or practice Yoga today? YES NO

Date: _____ Mon Tue Wed Thu Fri Sat Sun

Quote of the Day:

> "Life begins where fear ends."
> - Bhagwan Shree Rajneesh

Your Mood Today

Stress Level: 0 1 2 3 4 5 6 7 8 9 10
No Stress — Full Stress

Sleep Quality: 0 1 2 3 4 5 6 7 8 9 10
Very bad — Very well

How long did you sleep last night? _____ Hrs.

Time	Meals Taken Today	Symptoms Experienced:	How intense? (1: low, 5: severe)
	Breakfast:		
	Lunch:		
	Dinner:		
	Snacks:		

Bowel Movement:

How many liquid bowel movements you had today?

| One: | Two: | Three: | Four: | More than 4: |

Did you have any of the followings today?

Bowel Urgency: YES NO
Bleeding: YES NO
Partial evacuation: YES NO
Sinking defecation: YES NO

Mucus in the stool: YES NO
Painful bowel movement: YES NO
High pressure evacuation: YES NO
Other Symptoms: YES NO

Stool Type:

1. Very constipated: YES NO
2. Constipated: YES NO
3. Normal sausage-like: YES NO
4. Normal smooth: YES NO

5. Soft blobs: YES NO
6. Mushy: YES NO
7. Liquid: YES NO
Any Notes:

Activities:

Did you have a workout today? YES NO
Was it intense? YES NO
How long did you have workout? _____ Min.
Your weight changed today? YES NO
Did you have a good appetite? YES NO
How many glasses of water did you have? _____
Did you have time to meditate or practice Yoga today? YES NO

Date: _____   Mon Tue Wed Thu Fri Sat Sun
                 ○   ○   ○   ○   ○   ○   ○

Quote of the Day:

"The past is already gone; the future is not yet here. There's only one moment for you to live."
- Buddha

Your Mood Today [ ] [ ] [ ] [ ] [ ] [ ]

Stress Level: 0 1 2 3 4 5 6 7 8 9 10
No Stress   Full Stress

Sleep Quality: 0 1 2 3 4 5 6 7 8 9 10
Very bad   Very well

How long did you sleep last night? _____ Hrs.

Time	Meals Taken Today	Symptoms Experienced:	How intense? (1: low, 5: severe)
	Breakfast:		
	Lunch:		
	Dinner:		
	Snacks:		

Bowel Movement:

How many liquid bowel movements you had today?

| One: | Two: | Three: | Four: | More than 4: |

Did you have any of the followings today?

Bowel Urgency: YES NO
Bleeding: YES NO
Partial evacuation: YES NO
Sinking defecation: YES NO

Mucus in the stool: YES NO
Painful bowel movement: YES NO
High pressure evacuation: YES NO
Other Symptoms: YES NO

Stool Type:

1. Very constipated: YES NO
2. Constipated: YES NO
3. Normal sausage-like: YES NO
4. Normal smooth: YES NO
5. Soft blobs: YES NO
6. Mushy: YES NO
7. Liquid: YES NO
Any Notes:

Activities:

Did you have a workout today? YES NO
Was it intense? YES NO
Your weight changed today? YES NO
How many glasses of water did you have? _____

How long did you have workout? _____ Min.
Did you have a good appetite? YES NO
Did you have time to meditate or practice Yoga today? YES NO

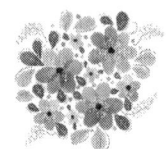

Week-3 IBS Control Record

Did you miss any activity due to your IBS condition?	YES NO
Do you think your IBS controlled well last week?	YES NO
Were you happy with your current treatment last week?	YES NO
Did you feel pain or discomfort last week?	YES NO
Did you have a good eating appetite last week?	YES NO
Did you feel fatigued last week?	YES NO
Did you feel depressed/anxious last week due to your IBS?	YES NO
Do you think you lost weight last week?	YES NO
Do you feel your bowel symptoms got better last week?	YES NO

Low FODMAP Diet Adherence:

Did you have any of the following foods this week?

Alcohol:	YES NO	Chocolate:	YES NO	Coffee:	YES NO
Soda:	YES NO	Sweet Fruits	YES NO	Lactose Products:	YES NO
Fatty/greasy Foods:	YES NO	Fried Foods:	YES NO	Gluten Products:	YES NO
FODMAP Sugars	YES NO	Raw Vegetables:	YES NO	Spicy Foods:	YES NO

Add any other suspicious foods you consumed: Did you get any discomfort?

1. _____ YES NO
2. _____ YES NO
3. _____ YES NO
4. _____ YES NO
5. _____ YES NO
6. _____ YES NO
7. _____ YES NO
8. _____ YES NO
9. _____ YES NO
10. _____ YES NO

Others:

Medications/Supplements taken this week: _____

Tell a good thing that happened this week: _____
_____

Other Notes: _____
_____
_____
_____
_____

Date: _____ ◯ Mon ◯ Tue ◯ Wed ◯ Thu ◯ Fri ◯ Sat ◯ Sun

Quote of the Day:
"When you are content to be simply yourself and don't compare or compete, everyone will respect you." - Lao Tzu

Your Mood Today

Stress Level: 0 — 10 (No Stress — Full Stress)

Sleep Quality: 0 — 10 (Very bad — Very well)

How long did you sleep last night? _____ Hrs.

Time	Meals Taken Today	Symptoms Experienced:	How intense? (1: low, 5: severe)
	Breakfast:		
	Lunch:		
	Dinner:		
	Snacks:		

Bowel Movement:

How many liquid bowel movements you had today?
| One: | Two: | Three: | Four: | More than 4: |

Did you have any of the followings today?

Bowel Urgency: YES NO
Bleeding: YES NO
Partial evacuation: YES NO
Sinking defecation: YES NO

Mucus in the stool: YES NO
Painful bowel movement: YES NO
High pressure evacuation: YES NO
Other Symptoms: YES NO

Stool Type:

1. Very constipated: YES NO
2. Constipated: YES NO
3. Normal sausage-like: YES NO
4. Normal smooth: YES NO
5. Soft blobs: YES NO
6. Mushy: YES NO
7. Liquid: YES NO
Any Notes:

Activities:

Did you have a workout today? YES NO
Was it intense? YES NO
How long did you have workout? ____ Min.
Your weight changed today? YES NO
Did you have a good appetite? YES NO
How many glasses of water did you have? _____
Did you have time to meditate or practice Yoga today? YES NO

Date: _____ ○ Mon ○ Tue ○ Wed ○ Thu ○ Fri ○ Sat ○ Sun

Quote of the Day:
> "The hardest thing of all is to find a black cat in a dark room, especially if there is no cat!"
> - Confucius

Your Mood Today [ ][ ][ ][ ][ ][ ]

Stress Level: [0 — 10] No Stress — Full Stress

Sleep Quality: [0 — 10] Very bad — Very well

How long did you sleep last night? _____ Hrs.

Time	Meals Taken Today	Symptoms Experienced:	How intense? (1: low, 5: severe)
	Breakfast:		
	Lunch:		
	Dinner:		
	Snacks:		

Bowel Movement:

How many liquid bowel movements you had today?
| One: | Two: | Three: | Four: | More than 4: |

Did you have any of the followings today?

Bowel Urgency: YES NO
Bleeding: YES NO
Partial evacuation: YES NO
Sinking defecation: YES NO

Mucus in the stool: YES NO
Painful bowel movement: YES NO
High pressure evacuation: YES NO
Other Symptoms: YES NO

Stool Type:

1. Very constipated: YES NO
2. Constipated: YES NO
3. Normal sausage-like: YES NO
4. Normal smooth: YES NO

5. Soft blobs: YES NO
6. Mushy: YES NO
7. Liquid: YES NO
Any Notes:

Activities:

Did you have a workout today? YES NO
Was it intense? YES NO
How long did you have workout? _____ Min.
Your weight changed today? YES NO
Did you have a good appetite? YES NO
How many glasses of water did you have? _____
Did you have time to meditate or practice Yoga today? YES NO

Date: _____ ○ Mon ○ Tue ○ Wed ○ Thu ○ Fri ○ Sat ○ Sun

Quote of the Day:
"If your eyes are blinded with your worries, you cannot see the beauty of the sunset."
— Jiddu Krishnamurti

Your Mood Today: 😊 🙂 😐 🙁 ☹️ 😣

Stress Level: 0 — 10 (No Stress — Full Stress)

Sleep Quality: 0 — 10 (Very bad — Very well)

How long did you sleep last night? _____ Hrs.

Time	Meals Taken Today	Symptoms Experienced:	How intense? (1: low, 5: severe)
	Breakfast:		
	Lunch:		
	Dinner:		
	Snacks:		

Bowel Movement:

How many liquid bowel movements you had today?
| One: | Two: | Three: | Four: | More than 4: |

Did you have any of the followings today?

Bowel Urgency: YES NO
Bleeding: YES NO
Partial evacuation: YES NO
Sinking defecation: YES NO

Mucus in the stool: YES NO
Painful bowel movement: YES NO
High pressure evacuation: YES NO
Other Symptoms: YES NO

Stool Type:

1. Very constipated: YES NO
2. Constipated: YES NO
3. Normal sausage-like: YES NO
4. Normal smooth: YES NO
5. Soft blobs: YES NO
6. Mushy: YES NO
7. Liquid: YES NO
Any Notes:

Activities:

Did you have a workout today? YES NO
Was it intense? YES NO
How long did you have workout? _____ Min.
Your weight changed today? YES NO
Did you have a good appetite? YES NO
How many glasses of water did you have? _____
Did you have time to meditate or practice Yoga today? YES NO

Date: _____   Mon Tue Wed Thu Fri Sat Sun

Quote of the Day:
> "The past is fog on our minds. The future? A complete dream. We can't neither guess the future, neither change the past." - Shams Tabrizi

Your Mood Today | | | | | |

Stress Level:
0 1 2 3 4 5 6 7 8 9 10
No Stress   Full Stress

Sleep Quality:
0 1 2 3 4 5 6 7 8 9 10
Very bad   Very well

How long did you sleep last night? _____ Hrs.

Time	Meals Taken Today	Symptoms Experienced:	How intense? (1: low, 5: severe)
	Breakfast:		
	Lunch:		
	Dinner:		
	Snacks:		

Bowel Movement:

How many liquid bowel movements you had today?
One: ▮ Two: ▮ Three: ▮ Four: ▮ More than 4: ▮

Did you have any of the followings today?

Bowel Urgency: YES NO
Bleeding: YES NO
Partial evacuation: YES NO
Sinking defecation: YES NO

Mucus in the stool: YES NO
Painful bowel movement: YES NO
High pressure evacuation: YES NO
Other Symptoms: YES NO

Stool Type:

1. Very constipated: YES NO
2. Constipated: YES NO
3. Normal sausage-like: YES NO
4. Normal smooth: YES NO
5. Soft blobs: YES NO
6. Mushy: YES NO
7. Liquid: YES NO
Any Notes:

Activities:

Did you have a workout today? YES NO
Was it intense? YES NO
Your weight changed today? YES NO
How many glasses of water did you have? _____

How long did you have workout? _____ Min.
Did you have a good appetite? YES NO
Did you have time to meditate or practice Yoga today? YES NO

Date: _____   *Mon Tue Wed Thu Fri Sat Sun*
              ○   ○   ○   ○   ○   ○   ○

Quote of the Day:
> "Fall seven times, stand up eight."
> - Japanese Proverb

Your Mood Today [😊][🙂][😐][🙁][☹️][😣]

Stress Level:
0 — 1 — 2 — 3 — 4 — 5 — 6 — 7 — 8 — 9 — 10
No Stress   Full Stress

Sleep Quality:
0 — 1 — 2 — 3 — 4 — 5 — 6 — 7 — 8 — 9 — 10
Very bad   Very well

How long did you sleep last night? _____ Hrs.

Time	Meals Taken Today	Symptoms Experienced:	How intense? (1: low, 5: severe)
	Breakfast:		
	Lunch:		
	Dinner:		
	Snacks:		

Bowel Movement:
How many liquid bowel movements you had today?
| One: | Two: | Three: | Four: | More than 4: |

Did you have any of the followings today?

Bowel Urgency: YES NO
Bleeding: YES NO
Partial evacuation: YES NO
Sinking defecation: YES NO

Mucus in the stool: YES NO
Painful bowel movement: YES NO
High pressure evacuation: YES NO
Other Symptoms: YES NO

Stool Type:

1. Very constipated: YES NO
2. Constipated: YES NO
3. Normal sausage-like: YES NO
4. Normal smooth: YES NO
5. Soft blobs: YES NO
6. Mushy: YES NO
7. Liquid: YES NO
Any Notes:

Activities:

Did you have a workout today? YES NO
Was it intense? YES NO
How long did you have workout? ____ Min.
Your weight changed today? YES NO
Did you have a good appetite? YES NO
How many glasses of water did you have? ____
Did you have time to meditate or practice Yoga today? YES NO

Date: _____   Mon Tue Wed Thu Fri Sat Sun

Quote of the Day:

> "Dance, when you're broken open. Dance, if you've torn the bandage off. Dance in the middle of the fighting. Dance in your blood. Dance when you're perfectly free." - Rumi

Your Mood Today

Stress Level: 0 1 2 3 4 5 6 7 8 9 10
No Stress — Full Stress

Sleep Quality: 0 1 2 3 4 5 6 7 8 9 10
Very bad — Very well

How long did you sleep last night? _____ Hrs.

Time	Meals Taken Today	Symptoms Experienced:	How intense? (1: low, 5: severe)
	Breakfast:		
	Lunch:		
	Dinner:		
	Snacks:		

Bowel Movement:

How many liquid bowel movements you had today?

One:	Two:	Three:	Four:	More than 4:

Did you have any of the followings today?

Bowel Urgency: YES NO
Bleeding: YES NO
Partial evacuation: YES NO
Sinking defecation: YES NO

Mucus in the stool: YES NO
Painful bowel movement: YES NO
High pressure evacuation: YES NO
Other Symptoms: YES NO

Stool Type:

1. Very constipated: YES NO
2. Constipated: YES NO
3. Normal sausage-like: YES NO
4. Normal smooth: YES NO
5. Soft blobs: YES NO
6. Mushy: YES NO
7. Liquid: YES NO
Any Notes:

Activities:

Did you have a workout today? YES NO
Was it intense? YES NO

How long did you have workout? ____ Min.

Your weight changed today? YES NO

Did you have a good appetite? YES NO

How many glasses of water did you have? _____

Did you have time to meditate or practice Yoga today? YES NO

Date: _____   Mon Tue Wed Thu Fri Sat Sun

Quote of the Day:

> "Be realistic: Plan for a miracle."
> - Osho

Your Mood Today

Stress Level: 0 — 10 (No Stress — Full Stress)

Sleep Quality: 0 — 10 (Very bad — Very well)

How long did you sleep last night? _____ Hrs.

Time	Meals Taken Today	Symptoms Experienced:	How intense? (1: low, 5: severe)
	Breakfast:		
	Lunch:		
	Dinner:		
	Snacks:		

Bowel Movement:

How many liquid bowel movements you had today?

| One: | Two: | Three: | Four: | More than 4: |

Did you have any of the followings today?

Bowel Urgency: YES NO
Bleeding: YES NO
Partial evacuation: YES NO
Sinking defecation: YES NO

Mucus in the stool: YES NO
Painful bowel movement: YES NO
High pressure evacuation: YES NO
Other Symptoms: YES NO

Stool Type:

1. Very constipated: YES NO
2. Constipated: YES NO
3. Normal sausage-like: YES NO
4. Normal smooth: YES NO
5. Soft blobs: YES NO
6. Mushy: YES NO
7. Liquid: YES NO

Any Notes:

Activities:

Did you have a workout today? YES NO
Was it intense? YES NO
Your weight changed today? YES NO
How many glasses of water did you have? _____

How long did you have workout? _____ Min.
Did you have a good appetite? YES NO
Did you have time to meditate or practice Yoga today? YES NO

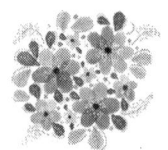

Week-4 IBS Control Record

Did you miss any activity due to your IBS condition?	YES NO
Do you think your IBS controlled well last week?	YES NO
Were you happy with your current treatment last week?	YES NO
Did you feel pain or discomfort last week?	YES NO
Did you have a good eating appetite last week?	YES NO
Did you feel fatigued last week?	YES NO
Did you feel depressed/anxious last week due to your IBS?	YES NO
Do you think you lost weight last week?	YES NO
Do you feel your bowel symptoms got better last week?	YES NO

Low FODMAO Diet Adherence:

Did you have any of the following foods this week?

Alcohol: YES NO	Chocolate: YES NO	Coffee: YES NO
Soda: YES NO	Sweet Fruits: YES NO	Lactose Products: YES NO
Fatty/greasy Foods: YES NO	Fried Foods: YES NO	Gluten Products: YES NO
FODMAP Sugars: YES NO	Raw Vegetables: YES NO	Spicy Foods: YES NO

Add any other suspicious foods you consumed: Did you get any discomfort?

1. _____ YES NO
2. _____ YES NO
3. _____ YES NO
4. _____ YES NO
5. _____ YES NO
6. _____ YES NO
7. _____ YES NO
8. _____ YES NO
9. _____ YES NO
10. _____ YES NO

Others:

Medications/Supplements taken this week: _____

Tell a good thing that happened this week: _____
_____

Other Notes: _____
_____
_____
_____
_____

Date: _____   Mon Tue Wed Thu Fri Sat Sun
                  ○   ○   ○   ○   ○   ○   ○

Quote of the Day:
"There are only two mistakes one can make along the road to truth; not going all the way, and not starting." - Buddha

Your Mood Today | 😊 | 🙂 | 😐 | 🙁 | ☹️ | 😖 |

Stress Level:
0 1 2 3 4 5 6 7 8 9 10
No Stress   Full Stress

Sleep Quality:
0 1 2 3 4 5 6 7 8 9 10
Very bad   Very well

How long did you sleep last night? _____ Hrs.

Time	Meals Taken Today	Symptoms Experienced:	How intense? (1: low, 5: severe)
	Breakfast:		
	Lunch:		
	Dinner:		
	Snacks:		

Bowel Movement:
How many liquid bowel movements you had today?
| One: | Two: | Three: | Four: | More than 4: |

Did you have any of the followings today?

Bowel Urgency: YES NO
Bleeding: YES NO
Partial evacuation: YES NO
Sinking defecation: YES NO

Mucus in the stool: YES NO
Painful bowel movement: YES NO
High pressure evacuation: YES NO
Other Symptoms: YES NO

Stool Type:

1. Very constipated: YES NO
2. Constipated: YES NO
3. Normal sausage-like: YES NO
4. Normal smooth: YES NO
5. Soft blobs: YES NO
6. Mushy: YES NO
7. Liquid: YES NO
Any Notes:

Activities:
Did you have a workout today? YES NO
Was it intense? YES NO
Your weight changed today? YES NO
How many glasses of water did you have? _____
How long did you have workout? ____ Min.
Did you have a good appetite? YES NO
Did you have time to meditate or practice Yoga today? YES NO

Date: _____   Mon Tue Wed Thu Fri Sat Sun
                  ○   ○   ○   ○   ○   ○   ○

Quote of the Day:

"Life is a series of natural and spontaneous changes. Don't resist them — that only creates sorrow. Let reality be the reality. Let things flow naturally forward in whatever way they like." - Lao Tzu

Your Mood Today [ ][ ][ ][ ][ ][ ]

Stress Level:
0 1 2 3 4 5 6 7 8 9 10
No Stress   Full Stress

Sleep Quality:
0 1 2 3 4 5 6 7 8 9 10
Very bad   Very well

How long did you sleep last night? _____ Hrs.

Time	Meals Taken Today	Symptoms Experienced:	How intense? (1: low, 5: severe)
	Breakfast:		
	Lunch:		
	Dinner:		
	Snacks:		

Bowel Movement:

How many liquid bowel movements you had today?

| One: | Two: | Three: | Four: | More than 4: |

Did you have any of the followings today?

Bowel Urgency: YES NO
Bleeding: YES NO
Partial evacuation: YES NO
Sinking defecation: YES NO

Mucus in the stool: YES NO
Painful bowel movement: YES NO
High pressure evacuation: YES NO
Other Symptoms: YES NO

Stool Type:

1. Very constipated: YES NO
2. Constipated: YES NO
3. Normal sausage-like: YES NO
4. Normal smooth: YES NO

5. Soft blobs: YES NO
6. Mushy: YES NO
7. Liquid: YES NO
Any Notes:

Activities:

Did you have a workout today? YES NO
Was it intense? YES NO
How long did you have workout? ____ Min.
Your weight changed today? YES NO
Did you have a good appetite? YES NO
How many glasses of water did you have? _____
Did you have time to meditate or practice Yoga today? YES NO

Date: _____   Mon Tue Wed Thu Fri Sat Sun

Quote of the Day:

> "A traveler without knowledge is a bird without wings."
> - Saadi

Your Mood Today

Stress Level: 0 – 10 (No Stress — Full Stress)

Sleep Quality: 0 – 10 (Very bad — Very well)

How long did you sleep last night? _____ Hrs.

Time	Meals Taken Today	Symptoms Experienced:	How intense? (1: low, 5: severe)
	Breakfast:		
	Lunch:		
	Dinner:		
	Snacks:		

Bowel Movement:

How many liquid bowel movements you had today?

| One: | Two: | Three: | Four: | More than 4: |

Did you have any of the followings today?

Bowel Urgency: YES NO
Bleeding: YES NO
Partial evacuation: YES NO
Sinking defecation: YES NO

Mucus in the stool: YES NO
Painful bowel movement: YES NO
High pressure evacuation: YES NO
Other Symptoms: YES NO

Stool Type:

1. Very constipated: YES NO
2. Constipated: YES NO
3. Normal sausage-like: YES NO
4. Normal smooth: YES NO
5. Soft blobs: YES NO
6. Mushy: YES NO
7. Liquid: YES NO
Any Notes:

Activities:

Did you have a workout today? YES NO
Was it intense? YES NO
Your weight changed today? YES NO
How many glasses of water did you have? _____

How long did you have workout? ____ Min.
Did you have a good appetite? YES NO
Did you have time to meditate or practice Yoga today? YES NO

Date: _____   Mon Tue Wed Thu Fri Sat Sun
                     ○   ○   ○   ○   ○   ○   ○

Quote of the Day:

> "Let go of your mind and then be mindful. Close your ears and listen!"
> - Rumi

Your Mood Today [😊] [🙂] [😐] [🙁] [😢]

Stress Level:
0 1 2 3 4 5 6 7 8 9 10
No Stress   Full Stress

Sleep Quality:
0 1 2 3 4 5 6 7 8 9 10
Very bad   Very well

How long did you sleep last night? _____ Hrs.

Time	Meals Taken Today	Symptoms Experienced:	How intense? (1: low, 5: severe)
	Breakfast:		
	Lunch:		
	Dinner:		
	Snacks:		

Bowel Movement:

How many liquid bowel movements you had today?

One:	Two:	Three:	Four:	More than 4:

Did you have any of the followings today?

Bowel Urgency: YES NO   Bleeding: YES NO   Partial evacuation: YES NO   Sinking defecation: YES NO

Mucus in the stool: YES NO   Painful bowel movement: YES NO   High pressure evacuation: YES NO   Other Symptoms: YES NO

Stool Type:

1. Very constipated: YES NO
2. Constipated: YES NO
3. Normal sausage-like: YES NO
4. Normal smooth: YES NO
5. Soft blobs: YES NO
6. Mushy: YES NO
7. Liquid: YES NO
Any Notes:

Activities:

Did you have a workout today? YES NO   Was it intense? YES NO

How long did you have workout? ____ Min.

Your weight changed today? YES NO

Did you have a good appetite? YES NO

How many glasses of water did you have? _____

Did you have time to meditate or practice Yoga today? YES NO

Date: _____   ○ Mon ○ Tue ○ Wed ○ Thu ○ Fri ○ Sat ○ Sun

Quote of the Day:
"Respect life, revere life. There is nothing more holy than life, nothing more divine than life."
- Osho

Your Mood Today [ ] [ ] [ ] [ ] [ ] [ ]

Stress Level: 0 1 2 3 4 5 6 7 8 9 10
No Stress   Full Stress

Sleep Quality: 0 1 2 3 4 5 6 7 8 9 10
Very bad   Very well

How long did you sleep last night? _____ Hrs.

Time	Meals Taken Today	Symptoms Experienced:	How intense? (1: low, 5: severe)
	Breakfast:		
	Lunch:		
	Dinner:		
	Snacks:		

Bowel Movement:
How many liquid bowel movements you had today?
| One: | Two: | Three: | Four: | More than 4: |

Did you have any of the followings today?

Bowel Urgency: YES NO
Bleeding: YES NO
Partial evacuation: YES NO
Sinking defecation: YES NO

Mucus in the stool: YES NO
Painful bowel movement: YES NO
High pressure evacuation: YES NO
Other Symptoms: YES NO

Stool Type:

1. Very constipated: YES NO
2. Constipated: YES NO
3. Normal sausage-like: YES NO
4. Normal smooth: YES NO

5. Soft blobs: YES NO
6. Mushy: YES NO
7. Liquid: YES NO
Any Notes:

Activities:

Did you have a workout today? YES NO
Was it intense? YES NO
Your weight changed today? YES NO
How many glasses of water did you have? _____

How long did you have workout? _____ Min.
Did you have a good appetite? YES NO
Did you have time to meditate or practice Yoga today? YES NO

Date: _____   Mon Tue Wed Thu Fri Sat Sun
                  ○   ○   ○   ○   ○   ○   ○

Quote of the Day:

> "If you find no one to support you on the spiritual path, walk alone. There is no companionship with the immature." - Buddha

Your Mood Today | | | | | | |

Stress Level:
0 1 2 3 4 5 6 7 8 9 10
No Stress   Full Stress

Sleep Quality:
0 1 2 3 4 5 6 7 8 9 10
Very bad   Very well

How long did you sleep last night? _____ Hrs.

Time	Meals Taken Today	Symptoms Experienced:	How intense? (1: low, 5: severe)
	Breakfast:		
	Lunch:		
	Dinner:		
	Snacks:		

Bowel Movement:

How many liquid bowel movements you had today?

One: ▢ Two: ▢ Three: ▢ Four: ▢ More than 4: ▢

Did you have any of the followings today?

Bowel Urgency: YES NO   Bleeding: YES NO   Partial evacuation: YES NO   Sinking defecation: YES NO
Mucus in the stool: YES NO   Painful bowel movement: YES NO   High pressure evacuation: YES NO   Other Symptoms: YES NO

Stool Type:

1. Very constipated: YES NO   2. Constipated: YES NO   3. Normal sausage-like: YES NO   4. Normal smooth: YES NO
5. Soft blobs: YES NO   6. Mushy: YES NO   7. Liquid: YES NO   Any Notes:

Activities:

Did you have a workout today? YES NO
Was it intense? YES NO
Your weight changed today? YES NO
How many glasses of water did you have? _____

How long did you have workout? _____ Min.
Did you have a good appetite? YES NO
Did you have time to meditate or practice Yoga today? YES NO

Date: _____   Mon Tue Wed Thu Fri Sat Sun

Quote of the Day:
> "In the midst of chaos, there is also opportunity."
> - Sun Tzu

Your Mood Today

Stress Level: 0 — 10 (No Stress — Full Stress)

Sleep Quality: 0 — 10 (Very bad — Very well)

How long did you sleep last night? _____ Hrs.

Time	Meals Taken Today	Symptoms Experienced:	How intense? (1: low, 5: severe)
	Breakfast:		
	Lunch:		
	Dinner:		
	Snacks:		

Bowel Movement:

How many liquid bowel movements you had today?

One:	Two:	Three:	Four:	More than 4:

Did you have any of the followings today?

- Bowel Urgency: YES / NO
- Bleeding: YES / NO
- Partial evacuation: YES / NO
- Sinking defecation: YES / NO
- Mucus in the stool: YES / NO
- Painful bowel movement: YES / NO
- High pressure evacuation: YES / NO
- Other Symptoms: YES / NO

Stool Type:

1. Very constipated: YES / NO
2. Constipated: YES / NO
3. Normal sausage-like: YES / NO
4. Normal smooth: YES / NO
5. Soft blobs: YES / NO
6. Mushy: YES / NO
7. Liquid: YES / NO
8. Any Notes:

Activities:

- Did you have a workout today? YES / NO
- Was it intense? YES / NO
- How long did you have workout? _____ Min.
- Your weight changed today? YES / NO
- Did you have a good appetite? YES / NO
- How many glasses of water did you have? _____
- Did you have time to meditate or practice Yoga today? YES / NO

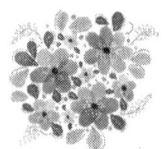

Week-5 IBS Control Record

Did you miss any activity due to your IBS condition?	YES NO
Do you think your IBS controlled well last week?	YES NO
Were you happy with your current treatment last week?	YES NO
Did you feel pain or discomfort last week?	YES NO
Did you have a good eating appetite last week?	YES NO
Did you feel fatigued last week?	YES NO
Did you feel depressed/anxious last week due to your IBS?	YES NO
Do you think you lost weight last week?	YES NO
Do you feel your bowel symptoms got better last week?	YES NO

Low FODMAP Diet Adherence:

Did you have any of the following foods this week?

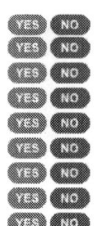

FODMAP

Alcohol: YES NO	Chocolate: YES NO	Coffee: YES NO
Soda: YES NO	Sweet Fruits: YES NO	Lactose Products: YES NO
Fatty/greasy Foods: YES NO	Fried Foods: YES NO	Gluten Products: YES NO
FODMAP Sugars: YES NO	Raw Vegetables: YES NO	Spicy Foods: YES NO

Add any other suspicious foods you consumed: Did you get any discomfort?

1. _____ YES NO
2. _____ YES NO
3. _____ YES NO
4. _____ YES NO
5. _____ YES NO
6. _____ YES NO
7. _____ YES NO
8. _____ YES NO
9. _____ YES NO
10. _____ YES NO

Others:

Medications/Supplements taken this week: _____

Tell a good thing that happened this week: _____

Other Notes: _____
_____
_____
_____
_____

Date: _____ Mon Tue Wed Thu Fri Sat Sun

Quote of the Day:
"The most important principle of the environment is that you are not the only element."
- Mahavira

Your Mood Today

Stress Level:
0 1 2 3 4 5 6 7 8 9 10
No Stress   Full Stress

Sleep Quality:
0 1 2 3 4 5 6 7 8 9 10
Very bad   Very well

How long did you sleep last night? _____ Hrs.

Time	Meals Taken Today	Symptoms Experienced:	How intense? (1: low, 5: severe)
	Breakfast:		
	Lunch:		
	Dinner:		
	Snacks:		

Bowel Movement:
How many liquid bowel movements you had today?

| One: | Two: | Three: | Four: | More than 4: |

Did you have any of the followings today?

Bowel Urgency: YES NO
Bleeding: YES NO
Partial evacuation: YES NO
Sinking defecation: YES NO

Mucus in the stool: YES NO
Painful bowel movement: YES NO
High pressure evacuation: YES NO
Other Symptoms: YES NO

Stool Type:

1. Very constipated: YES NO
2. Constipated: YES NO
3. Normal sausage-like: YES NO
4. Normal smooth: YES NO
5. Soft blobs: YES NO
6. Mushy: YES NO
7. Liquid: YES NO
Any Notes:

Activities:

Did you have a workout today? YES NO
Was it intense? YES NO
Your weight changed today? YES NO
How many glasses of water did you have? _____

How long did you have workout? ____ Min.
Did you have a good appetite? YES NO
Did you have time to meditate or practice Yoga today? YES NO

Date: _____   Mon Tue Wed Thu Fri Sat Sun

Quote of the Day:

"The heart has its own language. The heart knows a hundred thousand ways to speak."
- Rumi

Your Mood Today

Stress Level:

0 1 2 3 4 5 6 7 8 9 10
No Stress   Full Stress

Sleep Quality:

0 1 2 3 4 5 6 7 8 9 10
Very bad   Very well

How long did you sleep last night? _____ Hrs.

Time	Meals Taken Today	Symptoms Experienced:	How intense? (1: low, 5: severe)
	Breakfast:		
	Lunch:		
	Dinner:		
	Snacks:		

Bowel Movement:

How many liquid bowel movements you had today?

| One: | Two: | Three: | Four: | More than 4: |

Did you have any of the followings today?

Bowel Urgency: YES NO
Bleeding: YES NO
Partial evacuation: YES NO
Sinking defecation: YES NO

Mucus in the stool: YES NO
Painful bowel movement: YES NO
High pressure evacuation: YES NO
Other Symptoms: YES NO

Stool Type:

1. Very constipated: YES NO
2. Constipated: YES NO
3. Normal sausage-like: YES NO
4. Normal smooth: YES NO

5. Soft blobs: YES NO
6. Mushy: YES NO
7. Liquid: YES NO
Any Notes:

Activities:

Did you have a workout today? YES NO
Was it intense? YES NO

How long did you have workout? ____ Min.

Your weight changed today? YES NO

Did you have a good appetite? YES NO

How many glasses of water did you have? _____

Did you have time to meditate or practice Yoga today? YES NO

Date: _____   Mon Tue Wed Thu Fri Sat Sun

Quote of the Day:
> "Don't try to understand life. Live it! Don't try to understand love. Move into love. Then you will know, and that knowing will come out of your experience." - Osho

Your Mood Today

Stress Level: 0 — 10 (No Stress — Full Stress)

Sleep Quality: 0 — 10 (Very bad — Very well)

How long did you sleep last night? _____ Hrs.

Time	Meals Taken Today	Symptoms Experienced:	How intense? (1: low, 5: severe)
	Breakfast:		
	Lunch:		
	Dinner:		
	Snacks:		

Bowel Movement:

How many liquid bowel movements you had today?

One:	Two:	Three:	Four:	More than 4:

Did you have any of the followings today?

- Bowel Urgency: YES / NO
- Bleeding: YES / NO
- Partial evacuation: YES / NO
- Sinking defecation: YES / NO
- Mucus in the stool: YES / NO
- Painful bowel movement: YES / NO
- High pressure evacuation: YES / NO
- Other Symptoms: YES / NO

Stool Type:

1. Very constipated: YES / NO
2. Constipated: YES / NO
3. Normal sausage-like: YES / NO
4. Normal smooth: YES / NO
5. Soft blobs: YES / NO
6. Mushy: YES / NO
7. Liquid: YES / NO
8. Any Notes:

Activities:

- Did you have a workout today? YES / NO
- Was it intense? YES / NO
- Your weight changed today? YES / NO
- How many glasses of water did you have? _____
- How long did you have workout? ____ Min.
- Did you have a good appetite? YES / NO
- Did you have time to meditate or practice Yoga today? YES / NO

Date: _____   Mon Tue Wed Thu Fri Sat Sun

Quote of the Day:

"The key to growth is the introduction of higher dimensions of consciousness into our awareness."
- Lao Tzu

Your Mood Today

Stress Level: 0 1 2 3 4 5 6 7 8 9 10
No Stress — Full Stress

Sleep Quality: 0 1 2 3 4 5 6 7 8 9 10
Very bad — Very well

How long did you sleep last night? _____ Hrs.

Time	Meals Taken Today	Symptoms Experienced:	How intense? (1: low, 5: severe)
	Breakfast:		
	Lunch:		
	Dinner:		
	Snacks:		

Bowel Movement:

How many liquid bowel movements you had today?
One: Two: Three: Four: More than 4:

Did you have any of the followings today?

Bowel Urgency: YES NO
Bleeding: YES NO
Partial evacuation: YES NO
Sinking defecation: YES NO

Mucus in the stool: YES NO
Painful bowel movement: YES NO
High pressure evacuation: YES NO
Other Symptoms: YES NO

Stool Type:

1. Very constipated: YES NO
2. Constipated: YES NO
3. Normal sausage-like: YES NO
4. Normal smooth: YES NO

5. Soft blobs: YES NO
6. Mushy: YES NO
7. Liquid: YES NO
Any Notes:

Activities:

Did you have a workout today? YES NO
Was it intense? YES NO

How long did you have workout? ____ Min.

Your weight changed today? YES NO

Did you have a good appetite? YES NO

How many glasses of water did you have? _____

Did you have time to meditate or practice Yoga today? YES NO

Date: _____ ◯ Mon ◯ Tue ◯ Wed ◯ Thu ◯ Fri ◯ Sat ◯ Sun

Quote of the Day:
> "Make no friendship with an elephant keeper if you have no room to entertain an elephant!"
> - Saadi

Your Mood Today [😊] [🙂] [😐] [🙁] [☹️] [😣]

Stress Level: 0 — 10   No Stress .... Full Stress

Sleep Quality: 0 — 10   Very bad .... Very well

How long did you sleep last night? _____ Hrs.

Time	Meals Taken Today	Symptoms Experienced:	How intense? (1: low, 5: severe)
	Breakfast:		
	Lunch:		
	Dinner:		
	Snacks:		

Bowel Movement:
How many liquid bowel movements you had today?

| One: | Two: | Three: | Four: | More than 4: |

Did you have any of the followings today?

Bowel Urgency: YES NO
Bleeding: YES NO
Partial evacuation: YES NO
Sinking defecation: YES NO

Mucus in the stool: YES NO
Painful bowel movement: YES NO
High pressure evacuation: YES NO
Other Symptoms: YES NO

Stool Type:

1. Very constipated: YES NO
2. Constipated: YES NO
3. Normal sausage-like: YES NO
4. Normal smooth: YES NO
5. Soft blobs: YES NO
6. Mushy: YES NO
7. Liquid: YES NO
Any Notes:

Activities:

Did you have a workout today? YES NO
Was it intense? YES NO

How long did you have workout? ____ Min.

Your weight changed today? YES NO

Did you have a good appetite? YES NO

How many glasses of water did you have? _____

Did you have time to meditate or practice Yoga today? YES NO

Date: _____ Mon ○ Tue ○ Wed ○ Thu ○ Fri ○ Sat ○ Sun ○

Quote of the Day:

> "The secret of health for both mind and body is not to mourn for the past, worry about the future, or anticipate troubles, but to live in the present moment wisely and earnestly." - Buddha

Your Mood Today [ ] [ ] [ ] [ ] [ ] [ ]

Stress Level: 0 — 10 (No Stress — Full Stress)

Sleep Quality: 0 — 10 (Very bad — Very well)

How long did you sleep last night? _____ Hrs.

Time	Meals Taken Today	Symptoms Experienced:	How intense? (1: low, 5: severe)
	Breakfast:		
	Lunch:		
	Dinner:		
	Snacks:		

Bowel Movement:

How many liquid bowel movements you had today?

One:	Two:	Three:	Four:	More than 4:

Did you have any of the followings today?

- Bowel Urgency: YES / NO
- Bleeding: YES / NO
- Partial evacuation: YES / NO
- Sinking defecation: YES / NO
- Mucus in the stool: YES / NO
- Painful bowel movement: YES / NO
- High pressure evacuation: YES / NO
- Other Symptoms: YES / NO

Stool Type:

- 1. Very constipated: YES / NO
- 2. Constipated: YES / NO
- 3. Normal sausage-like: YES / NO
- 4. Normal smooth: YES / NO
- 5. Soft blobs: YES / NO
- 6. Mushy: YES / NO
- 7. Liquid: YES / NO
- Any Notes:

Activities:

- Did you have a workout today? YES / NO Was it intense? YES / NO
- How long did you have workout? _____ Min.
- Your weight changed today? YES / NO
- Did you have a good appetite? YES / NO
- How many glasses of water did you have? _____
- Did you have time to meditate or practice Yoga today? YES / NO

Date: _____   ○ Mon ○ Tue ○ Wed ○ Thu ○ Fri ○ Sat ○ Sun

Quote of the Day:
> "Don't be satisfied with stories, how things have gone with others. Unfold your own myth."
> - Rumi

Your Mood Today [ ] [ ] [ ] [ ] [ ] [ ]

Stress Level:
0 — 10 (No Stress — Full Stress)

Sleep Quality:
0 — 10 (Very bad — Very well)

How long did you sleep last night? _____ Hrs.

Time	Meals Taken Today	Symptoms Experienced:	How intense? (1: low, 5: severe)
	Breakfast:		
	Lunch:		
	Dinner:		
	Snacks:		

Bowel Movement:
How many liquid bowel movements you had today?

| One: | Two: | Three: | Four: | More than 4: |

Did you have any of the followings today?

Bowel Urgency: YES NO
Bleeding: YES NO
Partial evacuation: YES NO
Sinking defecation: YES NO

Mucus in the stool: YES NO
Painful bowel movement: YES NO
High pressure evacuation: YES NO
Other Symptoms: YES NO

Stool Type:

1. Very constipated: YES NO
2. Constipated: YES NO
3. Normal sausage-like: YES NO
4. Normal smooth: YES NO
5. Soft blobs: YES NO
6. Mushy: YES NO
7. Liquid: YES NO
Any Notes:

Activities:

Did you have a workout today? YES NO
Was it intense? YES NO
Your weight changed today? YES NO
How many glasses of water did you have? _____

How long did you have workout? _____ Min.
Did you have a good appetite? YES NO
Did you have time to meditate or practice Yoga today? YES NO

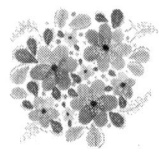

Week-6 IBS Control Record

Did you miss any activity due to your IBS condition? **YES** NO
Do you think your IBS controlled well last week? **YES** NO
Were you happy with your current treatment last week? **YES** NO
Did you feel pain or discomfort last week? **YES** NO
Did you have a good eating appetite last week? **YES** NO
Did you feel fatigued last week? **YES** NO
Did you feel depressed/anxious last week due to your IBS? **YES** NO
Do you think you lost weight last week? **YES** NO
Do you feel your bowel symptoms got better last week? **YES** NO

Low FODMAP Diet Adherence:

Did you have any of the following foods this week?

Alcohol: YES NO	Chocolate: YES NO	Coffee: YES NO
Soda: YES NO	Sweet Fruits: YES NO	Lactose Products: YES NO
Fatty/greasy Foods: YES NO	Fried Foods: YES NO	Gluten Products: YES NO
FODMAP Sugars: YES NO	Raw Vegetables: YES NO	Spicy Foods: YES NO

Add any other suspicious foods you consumed: Did you get any discomfort?

1. _____ YES NO
2. _____ YES NO
3. _____ YES NO
4. _____ YES NO
5. _____ YES NO
6. _____ YES NO
7. _____ YES NO
8. _____ YES NO
9. _____ YES NO
10. _____ YES NO

Others:

Medications/Supplements taken this week: _____

Tell a good thing that happened this week: _____

Other Notes: _____
_____
_____
_____
_____

Date: _____   Mon Tue Wed Thu Fri Sat Sun

Quote of the Day:
> "The ability to observe without evaluating is the highest form of intelligence."
> - Jiddu Krishnamurti

Your Mood Today

Stress Level:
0 — 10 (No Stress — Full Stress)

Sleep Quality:
0 — 10 (Very bad — Very well)

How long did you sleep last night? _____ Hrs.

Time	Meals Taken Today	Symptoms Experienced:	How intense? (1: low, 5: severe)
	Breakfast:		
	Lunch:		
	Dinner:		
	Snacks:		

Bowel Movement:

How many liquid bowel movements you had today?
One: Two: Three: Four: More than 4:

Did you have any of the followings today?

Bowel Urgency: YES NO
Bleeding: YES NO
Partial evacuation: YES NO
Sinking defecation: YES NO

Mucus in the stool: YES NO
Painful bowel movement: YES NO
High pressure evacuation: YES NO
Other Symptoms: YES NO

Stool Type:

1. Very constipated: YES NO
2. Constipated: YES NO
3. Normal sausage-like: YES NO
4. Normal smooth: YES NO
5. Soft blobs: YES NO
6. Mushy: YES NO
7. Liquid: YES NO
Any Notes:

Activities:

Did you have a workout today? YES NO
Was it intense? YES NO

How long did you have workout? ____ Min.

Your weight changed today? YES NO

Did you have a good appetite? YES NO

How many glasses of water did you have? _____

Did you have time to meditate or practice Yoga today? YES NO

Date: _____   Mon Tue Wed Thu Fri Sat Sun
                   ○   ○   ○   ○   ○   ○   ○

Quote of the Day:

> "The gem cannot be polished without friction, nor man perfected without trials."
> - Confucius

Your Mood Today | 😊 | 🙂 | 😐 | 🙁 | 😞 |

Stress Level:
0 1 2 3 4 5 6 7 8 9 10
No Stress   Full Stress

Sleep Quality:
0 1 2 3 4 5 6 7 8 9 10
Very bad   Very well

How long did you sleep last night? _____ Hrs.

Time	Meals Taken Today	Symptoms Experienced:	How intense? (1: low, 5: severe)
	Breakfast:		
	Lunch:		
	Dinner:		
	Snacks:		

Bowel Movement:

How many liquid bowel movements you had today?

| One: | Two: | Three: | Four: | More than 4: |

Did you have any of the followings today?

Bowel Urgency: Bleeding: Partial evacuation: Sinking defecation:
YES NO   YES NO   YES NO   YES NO

Mucus in the stool: Painful bowel movement: High pressure evacuation: Other Symptoms:
YES NO   YES NO   YES NO   YES NO

Stool Type:

1. Very constipated: 2. Constipated: 3. Normal sausage-like: 4. Normal smooth:
YES NO   YES NO   YES NO   YES NO

5. Soft blobs: 6. Mushy: 7. Liquid: Any Notes:
YES NO   YES NO   YES NO

Activities:

Did you have a workout today? YES NO
Was it intense? YES NO
Your weight changed today? YES NO
How many glasses of water did you have? _____

How long did you have workout? ____ Min.
Did you have a good appetite? YES NO
Did you have time to meditate or practice Yoga today? YES NO

Date: _____   Mon Tue Wed Thu Fri Sat Sun

Quote of the Day:
"To avoid disappointment, know what is sufficient. To avoid trouble, know when to stop. If you are able to do this, you will last a long time." - Lao Tzu

Your Mood Today

Stress Level:
0 1 2 3 4 5 6 7 8 9 10
No Stress   Full Stress

Sleep Quality:
0 1 2 3 4 5 6 7 8 9 10
Very bad   Very well

How long did you sleep last night? _____ Hrs.

Time	Meals Taken Today	Symptoms Experienced:	How intense? (1: low, 5: severe)
	Breakfast:		
	Lunch:		
	Dinner:		
	Snacks:		

Bowel Movement:
How many liquid bowel movements you had today?
One: Two: Three: Four: More than 4:

Did you have any of the followings today?

Bowel Urgency: Bleeding: Partial evacuation: Sinking defecation:
YES NO   YES NO   YES NO   YES NO

Mucus in the stool: Painful bowel movement: High pressure evacuation: Other Symptoms:
YES NO   YES NO   YES NO   YES NO

Stool Type:

1. Very constipated: 2. Constipated: 3. Normal sausage-like: 4. Normal smooth:
YES NO   YES NO   YES NO   YES NO

5. Soft blobs: 6. Mushy: 7. Liquid: Any Notes:
YES NO   YES NO   YES NO

Activities:

Did you have a workout today? YES NO
Was it intense? YES NO

How long did you have workout? _____ Min.

Your weight changed today? YES NO

How many glasses of water did you have?
_____

Did you have a good appetite? YES NO

Did you have time to meditate or practice Yoga today? YES NO

Date: _____ ○ Mon ○ Tue ○ Wed ○ Thu ○ Fri ○ Sat ○ Sun

Quote of the Day:
> "It is beautiful to be alone; it is also beautiful to be in love, to be with people. And they are complementary, not contradictory." - Osho

Your Mood Today | | | | | |

Stress Level:
0 1 2 3 4 5 6 7 8 9 10
No Stress — Full Stress

Sleep Quality:
0 1 2 3 4 5 6 7 8 9 10
Very bad — Very well

How long did you sleep last night? _____ Hrs.

Time	Meals Taken Today	Symptoms Experienced:	How intense? (1: low, 5: severe)
	Breakfast:		
	Lunch:		
	Dinner:		
	Snacks:		

Bowel Movement:
How many liquid bowel movements you had today?
One: ▢ Two: ▢ Three: ▢ Four: ▢ More than 4: ▢

Did you have any of the followings today?

Bowel Urgency: YES NO
Bleeding: YES NO
Partial evacuation: YES NO
Sinking defecation: YES NO

Mucus in the stool: YES NO
Painful bowel movement: YES NO
High pressure evacuation: YES NO
Other Symptoms: YES NO

Stool Type:

1. Very constipated: YES NO
2. Constipated: YES NO
3. Normal sausage-like: YES NO
4. Normal smooth: YES NO

5. Soft blobs: YES NO
6. Mushy: YES NO
7. Liquid: YES NO
Any Notes:

Activities:

Did you have a workout today? YES NO
Was it intense? YES NO

How long did you have workout? ____ Min.

Your weight changed today? YES NO

Did you have a good appetite? YES NO

How many glasses of water did you have? _____

Did you have time to meditate or practice Yoga today? YES NO

Date: _____   Mon Tue Wed Thu Fri Sat Sun

Quote of the Day:

> "All that we are is the result of what we have thought."
> - Buddha

Your Mood Today

Stress Level:
0 1 2 3 4 5 6 7 8 9 10
No Stress — Full Stress

Sleep Quality:
0 1 2 3 4 5 6 7 8 9 10
Very bad — Very well

How long did you sleep last night? _____ Hrs.

Time	Meals Taken Today	Symptoms Experienced:	How intense? (1: low, 5: severe)
	Breakfast:		
	Lunch:		
	Dinner:		
	Snacks:		

Bowel Movement:

How many liquid bowel movements you had today?

| One: | Two: | Three: | Four: | More than 4: |

Did you have any of the followings today?

Bowel Urgency: YES NO
Bleeding: YES NO
Partial evacuation: YES NO
Sinking defecation: YES NO

Mucus in the stool: YES NO
Painful bowel movement: YES NO
High pressure evacuation: YES NO
Other Symptoms: YES NO

Stool Type:

1. Very constipated: YES NO
2. Constipated: YES NO
3. Normal sausage-like: YES NO
4. Normal smooth: YES NO
5. Soft blobs: YES NO
6. Mushy: YES NO
7. Liquid: YES NO
Any Notes:

Activities:

Did you have a workout today? YES NO
Was it intense? YES NO

How long did you have workout? ____ Min.

Your weight changed today? YES NO

Did you have a good appetite? YES NO

How many glasses of water did you have? _____

Did you have time to meditate or practice Yoga today? YES NO

Date: _____ Mon Tue Wed Thu Fri Sat Sun

Quote of the Day:

> "Every leaf of the tree becomes a page of the book, once the heart is opened and it has learned to read." - Saadi

Your Mood Today

Stress Level:
0 1 2 3 4 5 6 7 8 9 10
No Stress — Full Stress

Sleep Quality:
0 1 2 3 4 5 6 7 8 9 10
Very bad — Very well

How long did you sleep last night? _____ Hrs.

Time	Meals Taken Today	Symptoms Experienced:	How intense? (1: low, 5: severe)
	Breakfast:		
	Lunch:		
	Dinner:		
	Snacks:		

Bowel Movement:

How many liquid bowel movements you had today?
One: ☐ Two: ☐ Three: ☐ Four: ☐ More than 4: ☐

Did you have any of the followings today?

Bowel Urgency: YES NO   Bleeding: YES NO   Partial evacuation: YES NO   Sinking defecation: YES NO

Mucus in the stool: YES NO   Painful bowel movement: YES NO   High pressure evacuation: YES NO   Other Symptoms: YES NO

Stool Type:

1. Very constipated: YES NO   2. Constipated: YES NO   3. Normal sausage-like: YES NO   4. Normal smooth: YES NO

5. Soft blobs: YES NO   6. Mushy: YES NO   7. Liquid: YES NO   Any Notes:

Activities:

Did you have a workout today? YES NO
Was it intense? YES NO

How long did you have workout? ____ Min.

Your weight changed today? YES NO

Did you have a good appetite? YES NO

How many glasses of water did you have? _____

Did you have time to meditate or practice Yoga today? YES NO

Date: _____   Mon Tue Wed Thu Fri Sat Sun

Quote of the Day:
"I have just three things to teach: simplicity, patience, compassion. These three are your greatest treasures." - Lao Tzu

Your Mood Today

Stress Level: 0 1 2 3 4 5 6 7 8 9 10
No Stress — Full Stress

Sleep Quality: 0 1 2 3 4 5 6 7 8 9 10
Very bad — Very well

How long did you sleep last night? _____ Hrs.

Time	Meals Taken Today	Symptoms Experienced:	How intense? (1: low, 5: severe)
	Breakfast:		
	Lunch:		
	Dinner:		
	Snacks:		

Bowel Movement:

How many liquid bowel movements you had today?

| One: | Two: | Three: | Four: | More than 4: |

Did you have any of the followings today?

Bowel Urgency: YES NO
Bleeding: YES NO
Partial evacuation: YES NO
Sinking defecation: YES NO

Mucus in the stool: YES NO
Painful bowel movement: YES NO
High pressure evacuation: YES NO
Other Symptoms: YES NO

Stool Type:

1. Very constipated: YES NO
2. Constipated: YES NO
3. Normal sausage-like: YES NO
4. Normal smooth: YES NO
5. Soft blobs: YES NO
6. Mushy: YES NO
7. Liquid: YES NO
Any Notes:

Activities:

Did you have a workout today? YES NO
Was it intense? YES NO

How long did you have workout? ____ Min.

Your weight changed today? YES NO

Did you have a good appetite? YES NO

How many glasses of water did you have? _____

Did you have time to meditate or practice Yoga today? YES NO

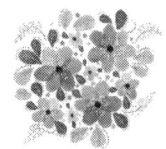

Week-7 IBS Control Record

Did you miss any activity due to your IBS condition?	YES NO
Do you think your IBS controlled well last week?	YES NO
Were you happy with your current treatment last week?	YES NO
Did you feel pain or discomfort last week?	YES NO
Did you have a good eating appetite last week?	YES NO
Did you feel fatigued last week?	YES NO
Did you feel depressed/anxious last week due to your IBS?	YES NO
Do you think you lost weight last week?	YES NO
Do you feel your bowel symptoms got better last week?	YES NO

Low FODMAP Diet Adherence:

Did you have any of the following foods this week?

Alcohol: YES NO	Chocolate: YES NO	Coffee: YES NO
Soda: YES NO	Sweet Fruits: YES NO	Lactose Products: YES NO
Fatty/greasy Foods: YES NO	Fried Foods: YES NO	Gluten Products: YES NO
FODMAP Sugars: YES NO	Raw Vegetables: YES NO	Spicy Foods: YES NO

Add any other suspicious foods you consumed: Did you get any discomfort?

1. _____ YES NO
2. _____ YES NO
3. _____ YES NO
4. _____ YES NO
5. _____ YES NO
6. _____ YES NO
7. _____ YES NO
8. _____ YES NO
9. _____ YES NO
10. _____ YES NO

Others:

Medications/Supplements taken this week: _____

Tell a good thing that happened this week: _____

Other Notes: _____

Date: _____   Mon Tue Wed Thu Fri Sat Sun

Quote of the Day:
> "Life is a balance of holding on and letting go."
> - Rumi

Your Mood Today

Stress Level: 0 — 10 (No Stress — Full Stress)

Sleep Quality: 0 — 10 (Very bad — Very well)

How long did you sleep last night? _____ Hrs.

Time	Meals Taken Today	Symptoms Experienced:	How intense? (1: low, 5: severe)
	Breakfast:		
	Lunch:		
	Dinner:		
	Snacks:		

Bowel Movement:
How many liquid bowel movements you had today?

One:	Two:	Three:	Four:	More than 4:

Did you have any of the followings today?

- Bowel Urgency: YES / NO
- Bleeding: YES / NO
- Partial evacuation: YES / NO
- Sinking defecation: YES / NO
- Mucus in the stool: YES / NO
- Painful bowel movement: YES / NO
- High pressure evacuation: YES / NO
- Other Symptoms: YES / NO

Stool Type:

1. Very constipated: YES / NO
2. Constipated: YES / NO
3. Normal sausage-like: YES / NO
4. Normal smooth: YES / NO
5. Soft blobs: YES / NO
6. Mushy: YES / NO
7. Liquid: YES / NO
8. Any Notes:

Activities:

- Did you have a workout today? YES / NO
- Was it intense? YES / NO
- How long did you have workout? ____ Min.
- Your weight changed today? YES / NO
- Did you have a good appetite? YES / NO
- How many glasses of water did you have? _____
- Did you have time to meditate or practice Yoga today? YES / NO

Date: _____   ◯ Mon ◯ Tue ◯ Wed ◯ Thu ◯ Fri ◯ Sat ◯ Sun

Quote of the Day:

> "Mind: A beautiful servant, a dangerous master."
> - Osho

Your Mood Today | 😀 | 🙂 | 😐 | 🙁 | 😞 | 😊 |

Stress Level:
0 1 2 3 4 5 6 7 8 9 10
No Stress — Full Stress

Sleep Quality:
0 1 2 3 4 5 6 7 8 9 10
Very bad — Very well

How long did you sleep last night? _____ Hrs.

Time	Meals Taken Today	Symptoms Experienced:	How intense? (1: low, 5: severe)
	Breakfast:		
	Lunch:		
	Dinner:		
	Snacks:		

Bowel Movement:
How many liquid bowel movements you had today?
| One: | Two: | Three: | Four: | More than 4: |

Did you have any of the followings today?

Bowel Urgency: YES NO
Bleeding: YES NO
Partial evacuation: YES NO
Sinking defecation: YES NO

Mucus in the stool: YES NO
Painful bowel movement: YES NO
High pressure evacuation: YES NO
Other Symptoms: YES NO

Stool Type:

1. Very constipated: YES NO
2. Constipated: YES NO
3. Normal sausage-like: YES NO
4. Normal smooth: YES NO
5. Soft blobs: YES NO
6. Mushy: YES NO
7. Liquid: YES NO
Any Notes:

Activities:

Did you have a workout today? YES NO
Was it intense? YES NO
How long did you have workout? ____ Min.
Your weight changed today? YES NO
Did you have a good appetite? YES NO
How many glasses of water did you have? _____
Did you have time to meditate or practice Yoga today? YES NO

Date: _____ Mon Tue Wed Thu Fri Sat Sun

Quote of the Day:
> "What you think, you become. What you feel, you attract. What you imagine you create."
> - Buddha

Your Mood Today | | | | | |

Stress Level:
0 1 2 3 4 5 6 7 8 9 10
No Stress — Full Stress

Sleep Quality:
0 1 2 3 4 5 6 7 8 9 10
Very bad — Very well

How long did you sleep last night? _____ Hrs.

Time	Meals Taken Today	Symptoms Experienced:	How intense? (1: low, 5: severe)
	Breakfast:		
	Lunch:		
	Dinner:		
	Snacks:		

Bowel Movement:
How many liquid bowel movements you had today?

| One: | Two: | Three: | Four: | More than 4: |

Did you have any of the followings today?

- Bowel Urgency: YES NO
- Bleeding: YES NO
- Partial evacuation: YES NO
- Sinking defecation: YES NO
- Mucus in the stool: YES NO
- Painful bowel movement: YES NO
- High pressure evacuation: YES NO
- Other Symptoms: YES NO

Stool Type:
1. Very constipated: YES NO
2. Constipated: YES NO
3. Normal sausage-like: YES NO
4. Normal smooth: YES NO
5. Soft blobs: YES NO
6. Mushy: YES NO
7. Liquid: YES NO
Any Notes:

Activities:
- Did you have a workout today? YES NO Was it intense? YES NO
- Your weight changed today? YES NO
- How many glasses of water did you have? _____
- How long did you have workout? _____ Min.
- Did you have a good appetite? YES NO
- Did you have time to meditate or practice Yoga today? YES NO

Date: _____   Mon Tue Wed Thu Fri Sat Sun

Quote of the Day:
> "Do the difficult things while they are easy and do the great things while they are small."
> - Lao Tzu

Your Mood Today

Stress Level:
0 1 2 3 4 5 6 7 8 9 10
No Stress — Full Stress

Sleep Quality:
0 1 2 3 4 5 6 7 8 9 10
Very bad — Very well

How long did you sleep last night? _____ Hrs.

Time	Meals Taken Today	Symptoms Experienced:	How intense? (1: low, 5: severe)
	Breakfast:		
	Lunch:		
	Dinner:		
	Snacks:		

Bowel Movement:

How many liquid bowel movements you had today?

| One: | Two: | Three: | Four: | More than 4: |

Did you have any of the followings today?

Bowel Urgency: YES NO
Bleeding: YES NO
Partial evacuation: YES NO
Sinking defecation: YES NO

Mucus in the stool: YES NO
Painful bowel movement: YES NO
High pressure evacuation: YES NO
Other Symptoms: YES NO

Stool Type:

1. Very constipated: YES NO
2. Constipated: YES NO
3. Normal sausage-like: YES NO
4. Normal smooth: YES NO
5. Soft blobs: YES NO
6. Mushy: YES NO
7. Liquid: YES NO

Any Notes:

Activities:

Did you have a workout today? YES NO
Was it intense? YES NO

How long did you have workout? _____ Min.

Your weight changed today? YES NO

Did you have a good appetite? YES NO

How many glasses of water did you have? _____

Did you have time to meditate or practice Yoga today? YES NO

Date: _____   Mon Tue Wed Thu Fri Sat Sun
                 ○   ○   ○   ○   ○   ○   ○

Quote of the Day:
"We can't change the direction of the wind, but we can adjust the sails."
- Indian Proverb

Your Mood Today | | | | | | |

Stress Level:
0 1 2 3 4 5 6 7 8 9 10
No Stress   Full Stress

Sleep Quality:
0 1 2 3 4 5 6 7 8 9 10
Very bad   Very well

How long did you sleep last night? _____ Hrs.

Time	Meals Taken Today	Symptoms Experienced:	How intense? (1: low, 5: severe)
	Breakfast:		
	Lunch:		
	Dinner:		
	Snacks:		

Bowel Movement:
How many liquid bowel movements you had today?

| One: | Two: | Three: | Four: | More than 4: |

Did you have any of the followings today?

Bowel Urgency: Bleeding: Partial evacuation: Sinking defecation:
YES NO   YES NO   YES NO   YES NO

Mucus in the stool: Painful bowel movement: High pressure evacuation: Other Symptoms:
YES NO   YES NO   YES NO   YES NO

Stool Type:

1. Very constipated: 2. Constipated: 3. Normal sausage-like: 4. Normal smooth:
YES NO   YES NO   YES NO   YES NO

5. Soft blobs: 6. Mushy: 7. Liquid: Any Notes:
YES NO   YES NO   YES NO

Activities:

Did you have a workout today? YES NO   How long did you have workout? ____ Min.
Was it intense? YES NO
Your weight changed today? YES NO   Did you have a good appetite? YES NO
How many glasses of water did you have?   Did you have time to meditate or practice Yoga today? YES NO
_____

Date: _____   Mon Tue Wed Thu Fri Sat Sun
                   ○   ○   ○   ○   ○   ○   ○

Quote of the Day:
> "If you are quiet enough, you will hear the flow of the universe. You will feel its rhythm. Go with this flow. Happiness lies ahead. Meditation is key." - Buddha

Your Mood Today | 😊 | 🙂 | 😐 | 🙁 | 😟 | 😠 |

Stress Level:
0 — 10 (No Stress — Full Stress)

Sleep Quality:
0 — 10 (Very bad — Very well)

How long did you sleep last night? _____ Hrs.

Time	Meals Taken Today	Symptoms Experienced:	How intense? (1: low, 5: severe)
	Breakfast:		
	Lunch:		
	Dinner:		
	Snacks:		

Bowel Movement:
How many liquid bowel movements you had today?
| One: | Two: | Three: | Four: | More than 4: |

Did you have any of the followings today?

Bowel Urgency: YES NO
Bleeding: YES NO
Partial evacuation: YES NO
Sinking defecation: YES NO

Mucus in the stool: YES NO
Painful bowel movement: YES NO
High pressure evacuation: YES NO
Other Symptoms: YES NO

Stool Type:

1. Very constipated: YES NO
2. Constipated: YES NO
3. Normal sausage-like: YES NO
4. Normal smooth: YES NO

5. Soft blobs: YES NO
6. Mushy: YES NO
7. Liquid: YES NO
Any Notes:

Activities:

Did you have a workout today? YES NO
Was it intense? YES NO
How long did you have workout? _____ Min.
Your weight changed today? YES NO
Did you have a good appetite? YES NO
How many glasses of water did you have? _____
Did you have time to meditate or practice Yoga today? YES NO

Date: _____   Mon Tue Wed Thu Fri Sat Sun

Quote of the Day:

> "He will win who knows when to fight and when not to fight."
> - Sun Tzu

Your Mood Today [ ] [ ] [ ] [ ] [ ] [ ]

Stress Level: 0 1 2 3 4 5 6 7 8 9 10
No Stress — Full Stress

Sleep Quality: 0 1 2 3 4 5 6 7 8 9 10
Very bad — Very well

How long did you sleep last night? _____ Hrs.

Time	Meals Taken Today	Symptoms Experienced:	How intense? (1: low, 5: severe)
	Breakfast:		
	Lunch:		
	Dinner:		
	Snacks:		

Bowel Movement:

How many liquid bowel movements you had today?

| One: | Two: | Three: | Four: | More than 4: |

Did you have any of the followings today?

- Bowel Urgency: YES / NO
- Bleeding: YES / NO
- Partial evacuation: YES / NO
- Sinking defecation: YES / NO
- Mucus in the stool: YES / NO
- Painful bowel movement: YES / NO
- High pressure evacuation: YES / NO
- Other Symptoms: YES / NO

Stool Type:

1. Very constipated: YES / NO
2. Constipated: YES / NO
3. Normal sausage-like: YES / NO
4. Normal smooth: YES / NO
5. Soft blobs: YES / NO
6. Mushy: YES / NO
7. Liquid: YES / NO

Any Notes:

Activities:

- Did you have a workout today? YES / NO Was it intense? YES / NO
- Your weight changed today? YES / NO
- How many glasses of water did you have? _____
- How long did you have workout? _____ Min.
- Did you have a good appetite? YES / NO
- Did you have time to meditate or practice Yoga today? YES / NO

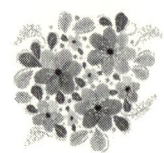

Week-8 IBS Control Record

Did you miss any activity due to your IBS condition?	YES NO
Do you think your IBS controlled well last week?	YES NO
Were you happy with your current treatment last week?	YES NO
Did you feel pain or discomfort last week?	YES NO
Did you have a good eating appetite last week?	YES NO
Did you feel fatigued last week?	YES NO
Did you feel depressed/anxious last week due to your IBS?	YES NO
Do you think you lost weight last week?	YES NO
Do you feel your bowel symptoms got better last week?	YES NO

Low FODMAP Diet Adherence:

Did you have any of the following foods this week?

Alcohol: YES NO	Chocolate: YES NO	Coffee: YES NO
Soda: YES NO	Sweet Fruits: YES NO	Lactose Products: YES NO
Fatty/greasy Foods: YES NO	Fried Foods: YES NO	Gluten Products: YES NO
FODMAP Sugars: YES NO	Raw Vegetables: YES NO	Spicy Foods: YES NO

Add any other suspicious foods you consumed: Did you get any discomfort?

1. _____ YES NO
2. _____ YES NO
3. _____ YES NO
4. _____ YES NO
5. _____ YES NO
6. _____ YES NO
7. _____ YES NO
8. _____ YES NO
9. _____ YES NO
10. _____ YES NO

Others:

Medications/Supplements taken this week: _____

Tell a good thing that happened this week: _____

Other Notes: _____

Date: _____   Mon Tue Wed Thu Fri Sat Sun

Quote of the Day:
"A lion chased me up a tree, and I greatly enjoyed the view from the top!"
- Confucius

Your Mood Today

Stress Level:
0 1 2 3 4 5 6 7 8 9 10
No Stress   Full Stress

Sleep Quality:
0 1 2 3 4 5 6 7 8 9 10
Very bad   Very well

How long did you sleep last night? _____ Hrs.

Time	Meals Taken Today	Symptoms Experienced:	How intense? (1: low, 5: severe)
	Breakfast:		
	Lunch:		
	Dinner:		
	Snacks:		

Bowel Movement:
How many liquid bowel movements you had today?

| One: | Two: | Three: | Four: | More than 4: |

Did you have any of the followings today?

Bowel Urgency: YES NO
Bleeding: YES NO
Partial evacuation: YES NO
Sinking defecation: YES NO

Mucus in the stool: YES NO
Painful bowel movement: YES NO
High pressure evacuation: YES NO
Other Symptoms: YES NO

Stool Type:

1. Very constipated: YES NO
2. Constipated: YES NO
3. Normal sausage-like: YES NO
4. Normal smooth: YES NO
5. Soft blobs: YES NO
6. Mushy: YES NO
7. Liquid: YES NO
Any Notes:

Activities:

Did you have a workout today? YES NO
Was it intense? YES NO
Your weight changed today? YES NO
How many glasses of water did you have? _____

How long did you have workout? ____ Min.
Did you have a good appetite? YES NO
Did you have time to meditate or practice Yoga today? YES NO

Date: _____   Mon Tue Wed Thu Fri Sat Sun
○ ○ ○ ○ ○ ○ ○

Quote of the Day:
> "Wherever you are, and whatever you do, be in love."
> - Rumi

Your Mood Today [ ][ ][ ][ ][ ]

Stress Level:
0 1 2 3 4 5 6 7 8 9 10
No Stress — Full Stress

Sleep Quality:
0 1 2 3 4 5 6 7 8 9 10
Very bad — Very well

How long did you sleep last night? _____ Hrs.

Time	Meals Taken Today	Symptoms Experienced:	How intense? (1: low, 5: severe)
	Breakfast:		
	Lunch:		
	Dinner:		
	Snacks:		

Bowel Movement:
How many liquid bowel movements you had today?
| One: | Two: | Three: | Four: | More than 4: |

Did you have any of the followings today?

Bowel Urgency: YES NO
Bleeding: YES NO
Partial evacuation: YES NO
Sinking defecation: YES NO

Mucus in the stool: YES NO
Painful bowel movement: YES NO
High pressure evacuation: YES NO
Other Symptoms: YES NO

Stool Type:

1. Very constipated: YES NO
2. Constipated: YES NO
3. Normal sausage-like: YES NO
4. Normal smooth: YES NO

5. Soft blobs: YES NO
6. Mushy: YES NO
7. Liquid: YES NO
Any Notes:

Activities:

Did you have a workout today? YES NO
Was it intense? YES NO

How long did you have workout? ____ Min.

Your weight changed today? YES NO

Did you have a good appetite? YES NO

How many glasses of water did you have? _____

Did you have time to meditate or practice Yoga today? YES NO

Date: _____ Mon Tue Wed Thu Fri Sat Sun

Quote of the Day:

> "Find ecstasy within yourself. It is not out there. It is in your innermost flowering. The one you are looking for is you." - Osho

Your Mood Today

Stress Level: 0 - 10 (No Stress — Full Stress)

Sleep Quality: 0 - 10 (Very bad — Very well)

How long did you sleep last night? _____ Hrs.

Time	Meals Taken Today	Symptoms Experienced:	How intense? (1: low, 5: severe)
	Breakfast:		
	Lunch:		
	Dinner:		
	Snacks:		

Bowel Movement:

How many liquid bowel movements you had today?

| One: | Two: | Three: | Four: | More than 4: |

Did you have any of the followings today?

- Bowel Urgency: YES NO
- Bleeding: YES NO
- Partial evacuation: YES NO
- Sinking defecation: YES NO
- Mucus in the stool: YES NO
- Painful bowel movement: YES NO
- High pressure evacuation: YES NO
- Other Symptoms: YES NO

Stool Type:

1. Very constipated: YES NO
2. Constipated: YES NO
3. Normal sausage-like: YES NO
4. Normal smooth: YES NO
5. Soft blobs: YES NO
6. Mushy: YES NO
7. Liquid: YES NO

Any Notes:

Activities:

- Did you have a workout today? YES NO
- Was it intense? YES NO
- Your weight changed today? YES NO
- How many glasses of water did you have? _____
- How long did you have workout? _____ Min.
- Did you have a good appetite? YES NO
- Did you have time to meditate or practice Yoga today? YES NO

Date: _____   Mon Tue Wed Thu Fri Sat Sun
                 ○   ○   ○   ○   ○   ○   ○

Quote of the Day:
"The whole secret of existence is to have no fear. Never fear what will become of you, depend on no one. Only the moment you reject all help is you freed." - Buddha

Your Mood Today

Stress Level: 0 – 10 (No Stress — Full Stress)

Sleep Quality: 0 – 10 (Very bad — Very well)

How long did you sleep last night? _____ Hrs.

Time	Meals Taken Today	Symptoms Experienced:	How intense? (1: low, 5: severe)
	Breakfast:		
	Lunch:		
	Dinner:		
	Snacks:		

Bowel Movement:

How many liquid bowel movements you had today?

| One: | Two: | Three: | Four: | More than 4: |

Did you have any of the followings today?

Bowel Urgency: YES NO   Bleeding: YES NO   Partial evacuation: YES NO   Sinking defecation: YES NO
Mucus in the stool: YES NO   Painful bowel movement: YES NO   High pressure evacuation: YES NO   Other Symptoms: YES NO

Stool Type:

1. Very constipated: YES NO   2. Constipated: YES NO   3. Normal sausage-like: YES NO   4. Normal smooth: YES NO
5. Soft blobs: YES NO   6. Mushy: YES NO   7. Liquid: YES NO   Any Notes:

Activities:

Did you have a workout today? YES NO   How long did you have workout? _____ Min.
Was it intense? YES NO
Your weight changed today? YES NO   Did you have a good appetite? YES NO
How many glasses of water did you have?   Did you have time to meditate or practice Yoga today? YES NO
_____

Date: _____   Mon Tue Wed Thu Fri Sat Sun

Quote of the Day:
> "For the wise man looks into space and he knows there are no limited dimensions."
> - Lao Tzu

Your Mood Today

<u>Stress Level:</u> 0 1 2 3 4 5 6 7 8 9 10
No Stress / Full Stress

<u>Sleep Quality:</u> 0 1 2 3 4 5 6 7 8 9 10
Very bad / Very well

How long did you sleep last night? _____ Hrs.

Time	Meals Taken Today	Symptoms Experienced:	How intense? (1: low, 5: severe)
	Breakfast:		
	Lunch:		
	Dinner:		
	Snacks:		

Bowel Movement:
How many liquid bowel movements you had today?

| One: | Two: | Three: | Four: | More than 4: |

Did you have any of the followings today?

Bowel Urgency: YES NO
Bleeding: YES NO
Partial evacuation: YES NO
Sinking defecation: YES NO

Mucus in the stool: YES NO
Painful bowel movement: YES NO
High pressure evacuation: YES NO
Other Symptoms: YES NO

Stool Type:
1. Very constipated: YES NO
2. Constipated: YES NO
3. Normal sausage-like: YES NO
4. Normal smooth: YES NO
5. Soft blobs: YES NO
6. Mushy: YES NO
7. Liquid: YES NO
Any Notes:

Activities:

Did you have a workout today? YES NO
Was it intense? YES NO
Your weight changed today? YES NO
How many glasses of water did you have? _____

How long did you have workout? _____ Min.
Did you have a good appetite? YES NO
Did you have time to meditate or practice Yoga today? YES NO

Date: _____   Mon Tue Wed Thu Fri Sat Sun
                  ○   ○   ○   ○   ○   ○   ○

Quote of the Day:
> "In the sea, there are countless treasures, but if you desire safety, it is on the shore."
> - Saadi

Your Mood Today | 😊 | 🙂 | 😐 | 🙁 | 😣 |

Stress Level: 0–10 (No Stress — Full Stress)

Sleep Quality: 0–10 (Very bad — Very well)

How long did you sleep last night? _____ Hrs.

Time	Meals Taken Today	Symptoms Experienced:	How intense? (1: low, 5: severe)
	Breakfast:		
	Lunch:		
	Dinner:		
	Snacks:		

Bowel Movement:

How many liquid bowel movements you had today?

| One: | Two: | Three: | Four: | More than 4: |

Did you have any of the followings today?

Bowel Urgency: YES NO
Bleeding: YES NO
Partial evacuation: YES NO
Sinking defecation: YES NO

Mucus in the stool: YES NO
Painful bowel movement: YES NO
High pressure evacuation: YES NO
Other Symptoms: YES NO

Stool Type:

1. Very constipated: YES NO
2. Constipated: YES NO
3. Normal sausage-like: YES NO
4. Normal smooth: YES NO
5. Soft blobs: YES NO
6. Mushy: YES NO
7. Liquid: YES NO

Any Notes:

Activities:

Did you have a workout today? YES NO
Was it intense? YES NO
Your weight changed today? YES NO
How many glasses of water did you have? _____

How long did you have workout? _____ Min.
Did you have a good appetite? YES NO
Did you have time to meditate or practice Yoga today? YES NO

Date: _____   Mon Tue Wed Thu Fri Sat Sun

Quote of the Day:

> "Wherever you go, east, west, north or south, think of it as a journey into yourself! The one who travels into itself travels the world." - Shams

Your Mood Today

Stress Level: 0 — 10 (No Stress — Full Stress)

Sleep Quality: 0 — 10 (Very bad — Very well)

How long did you sleep last night? _____ Hrs.

Time	Meals Taken Today	Symptoms Experienced:	How intense? (1: low, 5: severe)
	Breakfast:		
	Lunch:		
	Dinner:		
	Snacks:		

Bowel Movement:

How many liquid bowel movements you had today?

One:	Two:	Three:	Four:	More than 4:

Did you have any of the followings today?

- Bowel Urgency: YES NO
- Bleeding: YES NO
- Partial evacuation: YES NO
- Sinking defecation: YES NO
- Mucus in the stool: YES NO
- Painful bowel movement: YES NO
- High pressure evacuation: YES NO
- Other Symptoms: YES NO

Stool Type:

1. Very constipated: YES NO
2. Constipated: YES NO
3. Normal sausage-like: YES NO
4. Normal smooth: YES NO
5. Soft blobs: YES NO
6. Mushy: YES NO
7. Liquid: YES NO

Any Notes:

Activities:

- Did you have a workout today? YES NO Was it intense? YES NO
- Your weight changed today? YES NO
- How many glasses of water did you have? _____
- How long did you have workout? _____ Min.
- Did you have a good appetite? YES NO
- Did you have time to meditate or practice Yoga today? YES NO

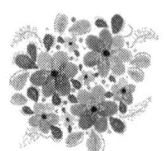

Week-9 IBS Control Record

Did you miss any activity due to your IBS condition? YES NO
Do you think your IBS controlled well last week? YES NO
Were you happy with your current treatment last week? YES NO
Did you feel pain or discomfort last week? YES NO
Did you have a good eating appetite last week? YES NO
Did you feel fatigued last week? YES NO
Did you feel depressed/anxious last week due to your IBS? YES NO
Do you think you lost weight last week? YES NO
Do you feel your bowel symptoms got better last week? YES NO

Low FODMAP Diet Adherence:

Did you have any of the following foods this week?

Alcohol: YES NO	Chocolate: YES NO	Coffee: YES NO
Soda: YES NO	Sweet Fruits: YES NO	Lactose Products: YES NO
Fatty/greasy Foods: YES NO	Fried Foods: YES NO	Gluten Products: YES NO
FODMAP Sugars: YES NO	Raw Vegetables: YES NO	Spicy Foods: YES NO

Add any other suspicious foods you consumed: Did you get any discomfort?

1. _____ YES NO
2. _____ YES NO
3. _____ YES NO
4. _____ YES NO
5. _____ YES NO
6. _____ YES NO
7. _____ YES NO
8. _____ YES NO
9. _____ YES NO
10. _____ YES NO

Others:

Medications/Supplements taken this week: _____

Tell a good thing that happened this week: _____

Other Notes: _____
_____
_____
_____

Date: _____ Mon Tue Wed Thu Fri Sat Sun

Quote of the Day:

> "Wear your ego like a loose-fitting garment."
> - Buddha

Your Mood Today

Stress Level:
0 1 2 3 4 5 6 7 8 9 10
No Stress — Full Stress

Sleep Quality:
0 1 2 3 4 5 6 7 8 9 10
Very bad — Very well

How long did you sleep last night? _____ Hrs.

Time	Meals Taken Today	Symptoms Experienced:	How intense? (1: low, 5: severe)
	Breakfast:		
	Lunch:		
	Dinner:		
	Snacks:		

Bowel Movement:

How many liquid bowel movements you had today?

| One: | Two: | Three: | Four: | More than 4: |

Did you have any of the followings today?

Bowel Urgency: YES NO   Bleeding: YES NO   Partial evacuation: YES NO   Sinking defecation: YES NO

Mucus in the stool: YES NO   Painful bowel movement: YES NO   High pressure evacuation: YES NO   Other Symptoms: YES NO

Stool Type:

1. Very constipated: YES NO
2. Constipated: YES NO
3. Normal sausage-like: YES NO
4. Normal smooth: YES NO
5. Soft blobs: YES NO
6. Mushy: YES NO
7. Liquid: YES NO
Any Notes:

Activities:

Did you have a workout today? YES NO
Was it intense? YES NO
Your weight changed today? YES NO
How many glasses of water did you have? ____

How long did you have workout? ____ Min.
Did you have a good appetite? YES NO
Did you have time to meditate or practice Yoga today? YES NO

Date: _____   Mon Tue Wed Thu Fri Sat Sun

Quote of the Day:

"Be a lotus flower. Be in the water, and do not let the water touch you."
- Osho

Your Mood Today

Stress Level:

0 1 2 3 4 5 6 7 8 9 10
No Stress   Full Stress

Sleep Quality:

0 1 2 3 4 5 6 7 8 9 10
Very bad   Very well

How long did you sleep last night? _____ Hrs.

Time	Meals Taken Today	Symptoms Experienced:	How intense? (1: low, 5: severe)
	Breakfast:		
	Lunch:		
	Dinner:		
	Snacks:		

Bowel Movement:

How many liquid bowel movements you had today?

| One: | Two: | Three: | Four: | More than 4: |

Did you have any of the followings today?

Bowel Urgency: YES NO
Bleeding: YES NO
Partial evacuation: YES NO
Sinking defecation: YES NO

Mucus in the stool: YES NO
Painful bowel movement: YES NO
High pressure evacuation: YES NO
Other Symptoms: YES NO

Stool Type:

1. Very constipated: YES NO
2. Constipated: YES NO
3. Normal sausage-like: YES NO
4. Normal smooth: YES NO

5. Soft blobs: YES NO
6. Mushy: YES NO
7. Liquid: YES NO
Any Notes:

Activities:

Did you have a workout today? YES NO
Was it intense? YES NO

How long did you have workout? ____ Min.

Your weight changed today? YES NO

Did you have a good appetite? YES NO

How many glasses of water did you have? _____

Did you have time to meditate or practice Yoga today? YES NO

Date: _____   Mon Tue Wed Thu Fri Sat Sun

Quote of the Day:

> "Let silence take you to the core of life."
> - Rumi

Your Mood Today | | | | | |

Stress Level:
0 1 2 3 4 5 6 7 8 9 10
No Stress — Full Stress

Sleep Quality:
0 1 2 3 4 5 6 7 8 9 10
Very bad — Very well

How long did you sleep last night? _____ Hrs.

Time	Meals Taken Today	Symptoms Experienced:	How intense? (1: low, 5: severe)
	Breakfast:		
	Lunch:		
	Dinner:		
	Snacks:		

Bowel Movement:

How many liquid bowel movements you had today?
One: ☐ Two: ☐ Three: ☐ Four: ☐ More than 4: ☐

Did you have any of the followings today?

Bowel Urgency: YES NO   Bleeding: YES NO   Partial evacuation: YES NO   Sinking defecation: YES NO
Mucus in the stool: YES NO   Painful bowel movement: YES NO   High pressure evacuation: YES NO   Other Symptoms: YES NO

Stool Type:

1. Very constipated: YES NO   2. Constipated: YES NO   3. Normal sausage-like: YES NO   4. Normal smooth: YES NO
5. Soft blobs: YES NO   6. Mushy: YES NO   7. Liquid: YES NO   Any Notes:

Activities:

Did you have a workout today? YES NO   Was it intense? YES NO
Your weight changed today? YES NO
How many glasses of water did you have? _____

How long did you have workout? _____ Min.
Did you have a good appetite? YES NO
Did you have time to meditate or practice Yoga today? YES NO

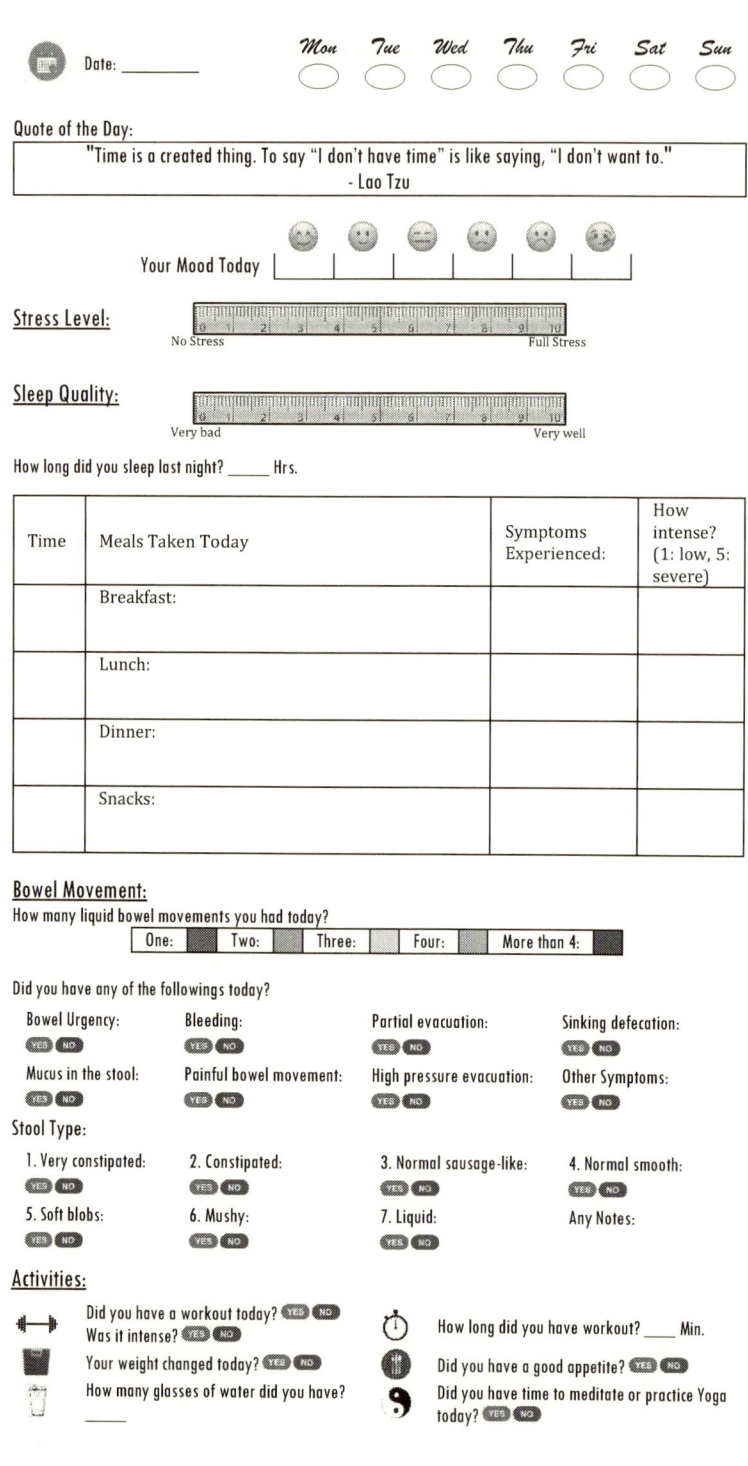

Date: _____   Mon Tue Wed Thu Fri Sat Sun
                 ○   ○   ○   ○   ○   ○   ○

Quote of the Day:
> "To compare is the very nature of a mind that is not awake to discover what is true."
> - Jiddu Krishnamurti

Your Mood Today | | | | | |

Stress Level:
0 1 2 3 4 5 6 7 8 9 10
No Stress   Full Stress

Sleep Quality:
0 1 2 3 4 5 6 7 8 9 10
Very bad   Very well

How long did you sleep last night? _____ Hrs.

Time	Meals Taken Today	Symptoms Experienced:	How intense? (1: low, 5: severe)
	Breakfast:		
	Lunch:		
	Dinner:		
	Snacks:		

Bowel Movement:
How many liquid bowel movements you had today?

| One: | Two: | Three: | Four: | More than 4: |

Did you have any of the followings today?

Bowel Urgency: YES NO
Bleeding: YES NO
Partial evacuation: YES NO
Sinking defecation: YES NO

Mucus in the stool: YES NO
Painful bowel movement: YES NO
High pressure evacuation: YES NO
Other Symptoms: YES NO

Stool Type:

1. Very constipated: YES NO
2. Constipated: YES NO
3. Normal sausage-like: YES NO
4. Normal smooth: YES NO
5. Soft blobs: YES NO
6. Mushy: YES NO
7. Liquid: YES NO
Any Notes:

Activities:

Did you have a workout today? YES NO
Was it intense? YES NO

Your weight changed today? YES NO

How many glasses of water did you have? _____

How long did you have workout? _____ Min.

Did you have a good appetite? YES NO

Did you have time to meditate or practice Yoga today? YES NO

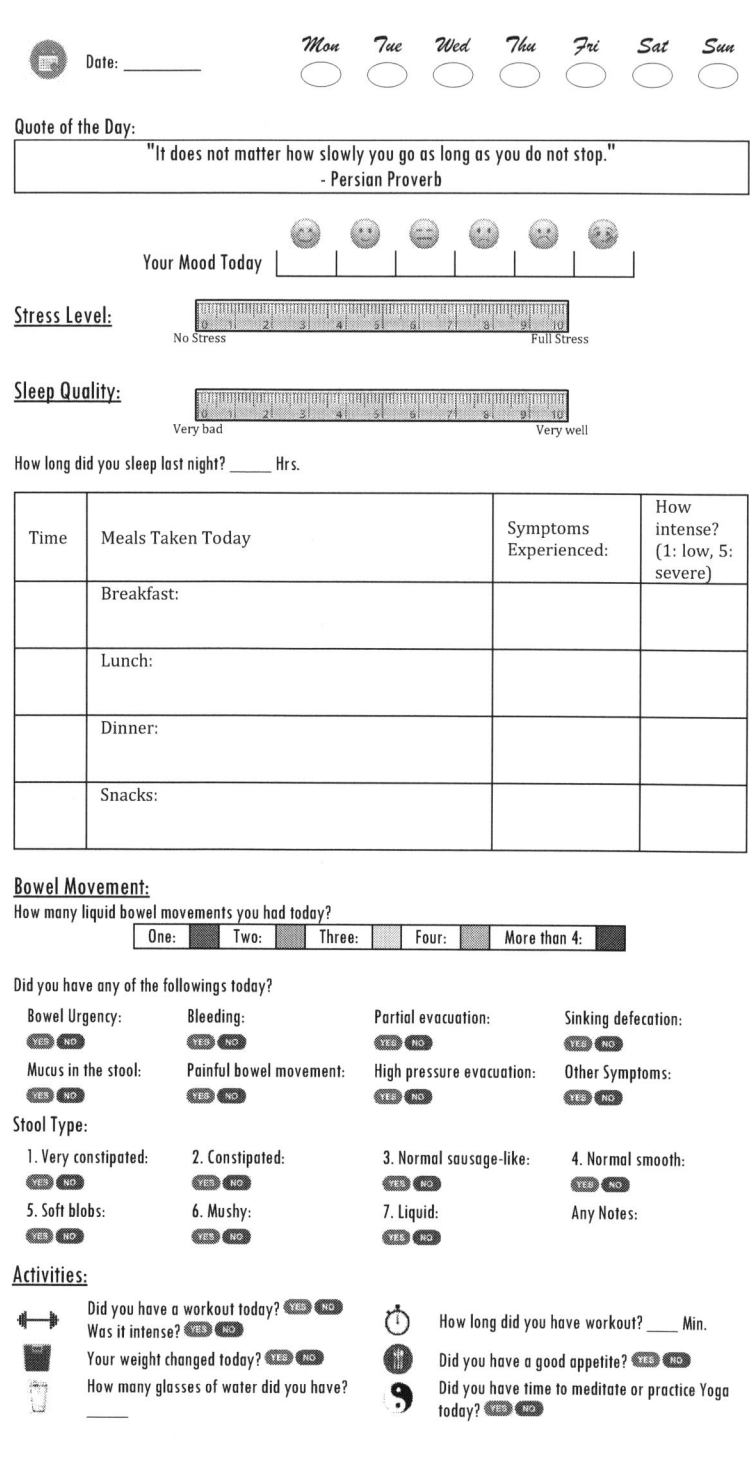

Date: _____   Mon Tue Wed Thu Fri Sat Sun

Quote of the Day:
> "Just as a snake sheds its skin, we must shed our past over and over again."
> — Buddha

Your Mood Today

Stress Level: 0 1 2 3 4 5 6 7 8 9 10
No Stress — Full Stress

Sleep Quality: 0 1 2 3 4 5 6 7 8 9 10
Very bad — Very well

How long did you sleep last night? _____ Hrs.

Time	Meals Taken Today	Symptoms Experienced:	How intense? (1: low, 5: severe)
	Breakfast:		
	Lunch:		
	Dinner:		
	Snacks:		

Bowel Movement:

How many liquid bowel movements you had today?

One:	Two:	Three:	Four:	More than 4:

Did you have any of the followings today?

- Bowel Urgency: YES NO
- Bleeding: YES NO
- Partial evacuation: YES NO
- Sinking defecation: YES NO
- Mucus in the stool: YES NO
- Painful bowel movement: YES NO
- High pressure evacuation: YES NO
- Other Symptoms: YES NO

Stool Type:

1. Very constipated: YES NO
2. Constipated: YES NO
3. Normal sausage-like: YES NO
4. Normal smooth: YES NO
5. Soft blobs: YES NO
6. Mushy: YES NO
7. Liquid: YES NO
   Any Notes:

Activities:

- Did you have a workout today? YES NO
- Was it intense? YES NO
- Your weight changed today? YES NO
- How many glasses of water did you have? _____
- How long did you have workout? _____ Min.
- Did you have a good appetite? YES NO
- Did you have time to meditate or practice Yoga today? YES NO

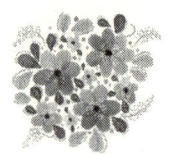

Week-10 IBS Control Record

Did you miss any activity due to your IBS condition?	YES NO
Do you think your IBS controlled well last week?	YES NO
Were you happy with your current treatment last week?	YES NO
Did you feel pain or discomfort last week?	YES NO
Did you have a good eating appetite last week?	YES NO
Did you feel fatigued last week?	YES NO
Did you feel depressed/anxious last week due to your IBS?	YES NO
Do you think you lost weight last week?	YES NO
Do you feel your bowel symptoms got better last week?	YES NO

Low FODMAP Diet Adherence:

Did you have any of the following foods this week?

Alcohol: YES NO	Chocolate: YES NO	Coffee: YES NO
Soda: YES NO	Sweet Fruits: YES NO	Lactose Products: YES NO
Fatty/greasy Foods: YES NO	Fried Foods: YES NO	Gluten Products: YES NO
FODMAP Sugars: YES NO	Raw Vegetables: YES NO	Spicy Foods: YES NO

Add any other suspicious foods you consumed: Did you get any discomfort?

1. _____ YES NO
2. _____ YES NO
3. _____ YES NO
4. _____ YES NO
5. _____ YES NO
6. _____ YES NO
7. _____ YES NO
8. _____ YES NO
9. _____ YES NO
10. _____ YES NO

Others:

Medications/Supplements taken this week: _____

Tell a good thing that happened this week: _____

Other Notes: _____
_____
_____
_____
_____

Date: _____   Mon Tue Wed Thu Fri Sat Sun

Quote of the Day:
"If you love a flower, don't pick it up. Because if you pick, it dies & it ceases to be what you love. So if you love a flower, let it be. Love is not about possession. Love is about appreciation." - Osho

Your Mood Today

Stress Level:
0 - No Stress ... 10 - Full Stress

Sleep Quality:
0 - Very bad ... 10 - Very well

How long did you sleep last night? _____ Hrs.

Time	Meals Taken Today	Symptoms Experienced:	How intense? (1: low, 5: severe)
	Breakfast:		
	Lunch:		
	Dinner:		
	Snacks:		

Bowel Movement:

How many liquid bowel movements you had today?

One:	Two:	Three:	Four:	More than 4:

Did you have any of the followings today?

Bowel Urgency: YES NO
Bleeding: YES NO
Partial evacuation: YES NO
Sinking defecation: YES NO

Mucus in the stool: YES NO
Painful bowel movement: YES NO
High pressure evacuation: YES NO
Other Symptoms: YES NO

Stool Type:

1. Very constipated: YES NO
2. Constipated: YES NO
3. Normal sausage-like: YES NO
4. Normal smooth: YES NO
5. Soft blobs: YES NO
6. Mushy: YES NO
7. Liquid: YES NO

Any Notes:

Activities:

Did you have a workout today? YES NO
Was it intense? YES NO
How long did you have workout? _____ Min.
Your weight changed today? YES NO
Did you have a good appetite? YES NO
How many glasses of water did you have? _____
Did you have time to meditate or practice Yoga today? YES NO

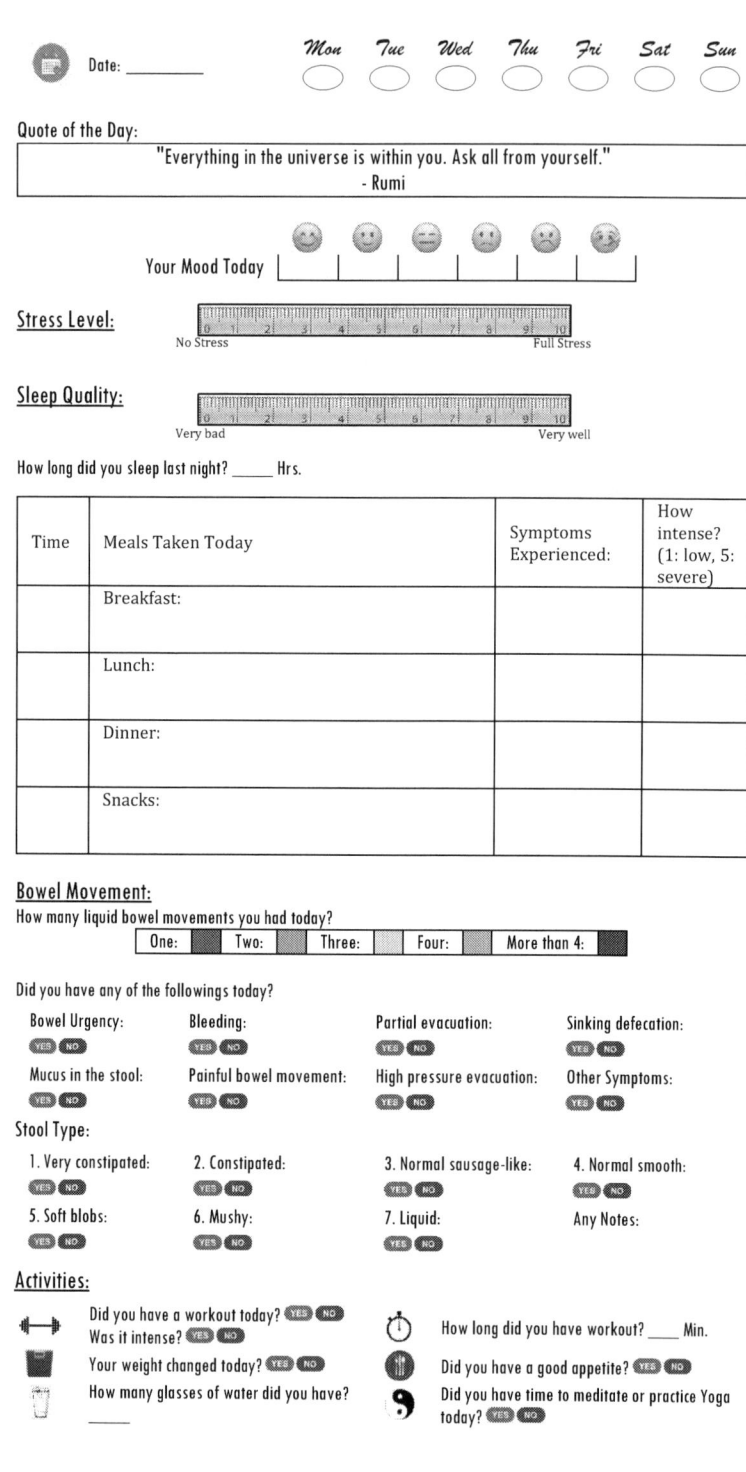

Date: _____   Mon Tue Wed Thu Fri Sat Sun

Quote of the Day:
"When there is silence, one finds the anchor of the universe within oneself."
- Lao Tzu

Your Mood Today

Stress Level:
0 1 2 3 4 5 6 7 8 9 10
No Stress   Full Stress

Sleep Quality:
0 1 2 3 4 5 6 7 8 9 10
Very bad   Very well

How long did you sleep last night? _____ Hrs.

Time	Meals Taken Today	Symptoms Experienced:	How intense? (1: low, 5: severe)
	Breakfast:		
	Lunch:		
	Dinner:		
	Snacks:		

Bowel Movement:
How many liquid bowel movements you had today?

| One: | Two: | Three: | Four: | More than 4: |

Did you have any of the followings today?

Bowel Urgency: YES NO
Bleeding: YES NO
Partial evacuation: YES NO
Sinking defecation: YES NO

Mucus in the stool: YES NO
Painful bowel movement: YES NO
High pressure evacuation: YES NO
Other Symptoms: YES NO

Stool Type:

1. Very constipated: YES NO
2. Constipated: YES NO
3. Normal sausage-like: YES NO
4. Normal smooth: YES NO
5. Soft blobs: YES NO
6. Mushy: YES NO
7. Liquid: YES NO
Any Notes:

Activities:

Did you have a workout today? YES NO
Was it intense? YES NO

Your weight changed today? YES NO

How many glasses of water did you have?
_____

How long did you have workout? ____ Min.

Did you have a good appetite? YES NO

Did you have time to meditate or practice Yoga today? YES NO

Date: _____ ○ Mon ○ Tue ○ Wed ○ Thu ○ Fri ○ Sat ○ Sun

Quote of the Day:

> "Before you embark on a journey of revenge, dig two graves."
> - Confucius

Your Mood Today: 😊 🙂 😐 🙁 😞 😣

Stress Level:
0 1 2 3 4 5 6 7 8 9 10
No Stress — Full Stress

Sleep Quality:
0 1 2 3 4 5 6 7 8 9 10
Very bad — Very well

How long did you sleep last night? _____ Hrs.

Time	Meals Taken Today	Symptoms Experienced:	How intense? (1: low, 5: severe)
	Breakfast:		
	Lunch:		
	Dinner:		
	Snacks:		

Bowel Movement:

How many liquid bowel movements you had today?

| One: | Two: | Three: | Four: | More than 4: |

Did you have any of the followings today?

Bowel Urgency: YES NO **Bleeding:** YES NO **Partial evacuation:** YES NO **Sinking defecation:** YES NO

Mucus in the stool: YES NO **Painful bowel movement:** YES NO **High pressure evacuation:** YES NO **Other Symptoms:** YES NO

Stool Type:

1. Very constipated: YES NO
2. Constipated: YES NO
3. Normal sausage-like: YES NO
4. Normal smooth: YES NO
5. Soft blobs: YES NO
6. Mushy: YES NO
7. Liquid: YES NO
Any Notes:

Activities:

Did you have a workout today? YES NO
Was it intense? YES NO
How long did you have workout? ____ Min.
Your weight changed today? YES NO
Did you have a good appetite? YES NO
How many glasses of water did you have? ____
Did you have time to meditate or practice Yoga today? YES NO

Date: _____   *Mon* *Tue* *Wed* *Thu* *Fri* *Sat* *Sun*

Quote of the Day:

> "On life's journey, faith is nourishment, virtuous deeds are a shelter, wisdom is the light by day, and right mindfulness is the protection by night. If a man lives a pure life, nothing can destroy him."
> - Buddha

Your Mood Today

Stress Level:
0 1 2 3 4 5 6 7 8 9 10
No Stress   Full Stress

Sleep Quality:
0 1 2 3 4 5 6 7 8 9 10
Very bad   Very well

How long did you sleep last night? _____ Hrs.

Time	Meals Taken Today	Symptoms Experienced:	How intense? (1: low, 5: severe)
	Breakfast:		
	Lunch:		
	Dinner:		
	Snacks:		

Bowel Movement:
How many liquid bowel movements you had today?
One: ▒   Two: ▒   Three: ▒   Four: ▒   More than 4: ▒

Did you have any of the followings today?

Bowel Urgency: YES NO
Bleeding: YES NO
Partial evacuation: YES NO
Sinking defecation: YES NO

Mucus in the stool: YES NO
Painful bowel movement: YES NO
High pressure evacuation: YES NO
Other Symptoms: YES NO

Stool Type:

1. Very constipated: YES NO
2. Constipated: YES NO
3. Normal sausage-like: YES NO
4. Normal smooth: YES NO

5. Soft blobs: YES NO
6. Mushy: YES NO
7. Liquid: YES NO
Any Notes:

Activities:

Did you have a workout today? YES NO
Was it intense? YES NO
Your weight changed today? YES NO
How many glasses of water did you have? _____

How long did you have workout? _____ Min.
Did you have a good appetite? YES NO
Did you have time to meditate or practice Yoga today? YES NO

Date: _____   Mon Tue Wed Thu Fri Sat Sun
                    ◯   ◯   ◯   ◯   ◯   ◯   ◯

Quote of the Day:

> "Tomorrow never comes; it is always today."
> - Osho

Your Mood Today [😀][🙂][😐][🙁][😣]

Stress Level: 0 1 2 3 4 5 6 7 8 9 10
                  No Stress   Full Stress

Sleep Quality: 0 1 2 3 4 5 6 7 8 9 10
                  Very bad   Very well

How long did you sleep last night? _____ Hrs.

Time	Meals Taken Today	Symptoms Experienced:	How intense? (1: low, 5: severe)
	Breakfast:		
	Lunch:		
	Dinner:		
	Snacks:		

Bowel Movement:

How many liquid bowel movements you had today?

| One: | Two: | Three: | Four: | More than 4: |

Did you have any of the followings today?

Bowel Urgency: YES NO   **Bleeding:** YES NO   **Partial evacuation:** YES NO   **Sinking defecation:** YES NO

Mucus in the stool: YES NO   **Painful bowel movement:** YES NO   **High pressure evacuation:** YES NO   **Other Symptoms:** YES NO

Stool Type:

1. Very constipated: YES NO   2. Constipated: YES NO   3. Normal sausage-like: YES NO   4. Normal smooth: YES NO
5. Soft blobs: YES NO   6. Mushy: YES NO   7. Liquid: YES NO   Any Notes:

Activities:

Did you have a workout today? YES NO   Was it intense? YES NO   How long did you have workout? ____ Min.

Your weight changed today? YES NO   Did you have a good appetite? YES NO

How many glasses of water did you have? _____   Did you have time to meditate or practice Yoga today? YES NO

Date: _____   Mon Tue Wed Thu Fri Sat Sun
                  ○   ○   ○   ○   ○   ○   ○

Quote of the Day:
"A wise man adapts himself to circumstances, as water shapes itself to the vessel that contains it."
- Chinese Proverb

Your Mood Today | | | | | | |

Stress Level:
0 1 2 3 4 5 6 7 8 9 10
No Stress   Full Stress

Sleep Quality:
0 1 2 3 4 5 6 7 8 9 10
Very bad   Very well

How long did you sleep last night? _____ Hrs.

Time	Meals Taken Today	Symptoms Experienced:	How intense? (1: low, 5: severe)
	Breakfast:		
	Lunch:		
	Dinner:		
	Snacks:		

Bowel Movement:
How many liquid bowel movements you had today?

One:	Two:	Three:	Four:	More than 4:

Did you have any of the followings today?

Bowel Urgency: YES NO
Bleeding: YES NO
Partial evacuation: YES NO
Sinking defecation: YES NO

Mucus in the stool: YES NO
Painful bowel movement: YES NO
High pressure evacuation: YES NO
Other Symptoms: YES NO

Stool Type:

1. Very constipated: YES NO
2. Constipated: YES NO
3. Normal sausage-like: YES NO
4. Normal smooth: YES NO
5. Soft blobs: YES NO
6. Mushy: YES NO
7. Liquid: YES NO
Any Notes:

Activities:

Did you have a workout today? YES NO
Was it intense? YES NO

How long did you have workout? ____ Min.

Your weight changed today? YES NO

Did you have a good appetite? YES NO

How many glasses of water did you have?
_____

Did you have time to meditate or practice Yoga today? YES NO

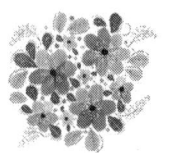

Week-11 IBS Control Record

Did you miss any activity due to your IBS condition? YES NO
Do you think your IBS controlled well last week? YES NO
Were you happy with your current treatment last week? YES NO
Did you feel pain or discomfort last week? YES NO
Did you have a good eating appetite last week? YES NO
Did you feel fatigued last week? YES NO
Did you feel depressed/anxious last week due to your IBS? YES NO
Do you think you lost weight last week? YES NO
Do you feel your bowel symptoms got better last week? YES NO

Low FODMAP Diet Adherence:

Did you have any of the following foods this week?

Alcohol: YES NO	Chocolate: YES NO	Coffee: YES NO
Soda: YES NO	Sweet Fruits: YES NO	Lactose Products: YES NO
Fatty/greasy Foods: YES NO	Fried Foods: YES NO	Gluten Products: YES NO
FODMAP Sugars: YES NO	Raw Vegetables: YES NO	Spicy Foods: YES NO

Add any other suspicious foods you consumed: Did you get any discomfort?

1. _____ YES NO
2. _____ YES NO
3. _____ YES NO
4. _____ YES NO
5. _____ YES NO
6. _____ YES NO
7. _____ YES NO
8. _____ YES NO
9. _____ YES NO
10. _____ YES NO

Others:

Medications/Supplements taken this week: _____

Tell a good thing that happened this week: _____

Other Notes: _____

Date: _____   Mon Tue Wed Thu Fri Sat Sun

Quote of the Day:
"If the problem can be solved, why worry? If the problem cannot be solved, worrying will do you no good." - Buddha

Your Mood Today

Stress Level:
0 1 2 3 4 5 6 7 8 9 10
No Stress — Full Stress

Sleep Quality:
0 1 2 3 4 5 6 7 8 9 10
Very bad — Very well

How long did you sleep last night? _____ Hrs.

Time	Meals Taken Today	Symptoms Experienced:	How intense? (1: low, 5: severe)
	Breakfast:		
	Lunch:		
	Dinner:		
	Snacks:		

Bowel Movement:
How many liquid bowel movements you had today?
| One: | Two: | Three: | Four: | More than 4: |

Did you have any of the followings today?

Bowel Urgency: YES NO
Bleeding: YES NO
Partial evacuation: YES NO
Sinking defecation: YES NO

Mucus in the stool: YES NO
Painful bowel movement: YES NO
High pressure evacuation: YES NO
Other Symptoms: YES NO

Stool Type:

1. Very constipated: YES NO
2. Constipated: YES NO
3. Normal sausage-like: YES NO
4. Normal smooth: YES NO
5. Soft blobs: YES NO
6. Mushy: YES NO
7. Liquid: YES NO
Any Notes:

Activities:

Did you have a workout today? YES NO
Was it intense? YES NO
Your weight changed today? YES NO
How many glasses of water did you have? _____

How long did you have workout? ____ Min.
Did you have a good appetite? YES NO
Did you have time to meditate or practice Yoga today? YES NO

Date: _____   Mon Tue Wed Thu Fri Sat Sun
                  ○   ○   ○   ○   ○   ○   ○

Quote of the Day:
> "You have seen your own strength. You have seen your own beauty. You have seen your golden wings. Why do you worry?" - Rumi

Your Mood Today [😊][🙂][😐][🙁][☹️][😢]

Stress Level:
0 1 2 3 4 5 6 7 8 9 10
No Stress   Full Stress

Sleep Quality:
0 1 2 3 4 5 6 7 8 9 10
Very bad   Very well

How long did you sleep last night? _____ Hrs.

Time	Meals Taken Today	Symptoms Experienced:	How intense? (1: low, 5: severe)
	Breakfast:		
	Lunch:		
	Dinner:		
	Snacks:		

Bowel Movement:
How many liquid bowel movements you had today?

| One: | Two: | Three: | Four: | More than 4: |

Did you have any of the followings today?

Bowel Urgency: YES NO   **Bleeding:** YES NO   **Partial evacuation:** YES NO   **Sinking defecation:** YES NO

Mucus in the stool: YES NO   **Painful bowel movement:** YES NO   **High pressure evacuation:** YES NO   **Other Symptoms:** YES NO

Stool Type:
1. Very constipated: YES NO
2. Constipated: YES NO
3. Normal sausage-like: YES NO
4. Normal smooth: YES NO
5. Soft blobs: YES NO
6. Mushy: YES NO
7. Liquid: YES NO
Any Notes:

Activities:
Did you have a workout today? YES NO
Was it intense? YES NO
Your weight changed today? YES NO
How many glasses of water did you have? _____

How long did you have workout? _____ Min.
Did you have a good appetite? YES NO
Did you have time to meditate or practice Yoga today? YES NO

Date: _____   Mon Tue Wed Thu Fri Sat Sun
○ ○ ○ ○ ○ ○ ○

Quote of the Day:
"What is discipline? Discipline means creating an order within you. As you are, you are a chaos."
- Osho

Your Mood Today | | | | | |

Stress Level:
0 1 2 3 4 5 6 7 8 9 10
No Stress — Full Stress

Sleep Quality:
0 1 2 3 4 5 6 7 8 9 10
Very bad — Very well

How long did you sleep last night? _____ Hrs.

Time	Meals Taken Today	Symptoms Experienced:	How intense? (1: low, 5: severe)
	Breakfast:		
	Lunch:		
	Dinner:		
	Snacks:		

Bowel Movement:
How many liquid bowel movements you had today?

One:	Two:	Three:	Four:	More than 4:

Did you have any of the followings today?

Bowel Urgency: YES NO
Bleeding: YES NO
Partial evacuation: YES NO
Sinking defecation: YES NO
Mucus in the stool: YES NO
Painful bowel movement: YES NO
High pressure evacuation: YES NO
Other Symptoms: YES NO

Stool Type:

1. Very constipated: YES NO
2. Constipated: YES NO
3. Normal sausage-like: YES NO
4. Normal smooth: YES NO
5. Soft blobs: YES NO
6. Mushy: YES NO
7. Liquid: YES NO
Any Notes:

Activities:
Did you have a workout today? YES NO
Was it intense? YES NO
Your weight changed today? YES NO
How many glasses of water did you have? _____
How long did you have workout? ____ Min.
Did you have a good appetite? YES NO
Did you have time to meditate or practice Yoga today? YES NO

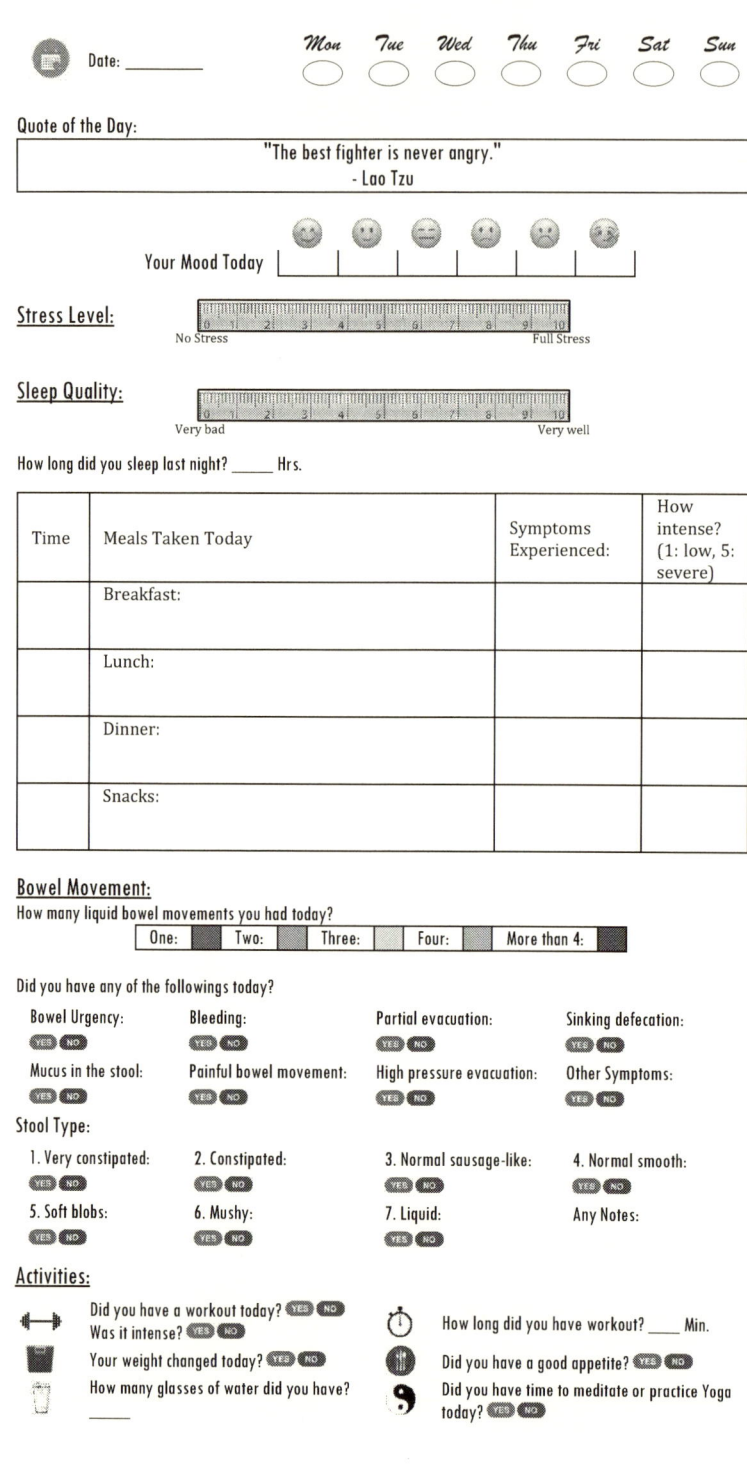

Date: _____   Mon Tue Wed Thu Fri Sat Sun
                  ○   ○   ○   ○   ○   ○   ○

Quote of the Day:
"As rain falls equally on the just and the unjust, do not burden your heart with judgments but rain your kindness equally on all." - Buddha

Your Mood Today | | | | | | |

Stress Level:
0 1 2 3 4 5 6 7 8 9 10
No Stress   Full Stress

Sleep Quality:
0 1 2 3 4 5 6 7 8 9 10
Very bad   Very well

How long did you sleep last night? _____ Hrs.

Time	Meals Taken Today	Symptoms Experienced:	How intense? (1: low, 5: severe)
	Breakfast:		
	Lunch:		
	Dinner:		
	Snacks:		

Bowel Movement:
How many liquid bowel movements you had today?
| One: | Two: | Three: | Four: | More than 4: |

Did you have any of the followings today?

Bowel Urgency: YES NO
Bleeding: YES NO
Partial evacuation: YES NO
Sinking defecation: YES NO

Mucus in the stool: YES NO
Painful bowel movement: YES NO
High pressure evacuation: YES NO
Other Symptoms: YES NO

Stool Type:
1. Very constipated: YES NO
2. Constipated: YES NO
3. Normal sausage-like: YES NO
4. Normal smooth: YES NO
5. Soft blobs: YES NO
6. Mushy: YES NO
7. Liquid: YES NO
Any Notes:

Activities:
Did you have a workout today? YES NO
Was it intense? YES NO
How long did you have workout? _____ Min.
Your weight changed today? YES NO
Did you have a good appetite? YES NO
How many glasses of water did you have? _____
Did you have time to meditate or practice Yoga today? YES NO

Date: _____   Mon Tue Wed Thu Fri Sat Sun

Quote of the Day:
> "On a day when the wind is perfect, the sail just needs to open, and the world is full of beauty. Today is such a day." - Rumi

Your Mood Today: [ ] [ ] [ ] [ ] [ ] [ ]

Stress Level: 0 1 2 3 4 5 6 7 8 9 10
No Stress — Full Stress

Sleep Quality: 0 1 2 3 4 5 6 7 8 9 10
Very bad — Very well

How long did you sleep last night? _____ Hrs.

Time	Meals Taken Today	Symptoms Experienced:	How intense? (1: low, 5: severe)
	Breakfast:		
	Lunch:		
	Dinner:		
	Snacks:		

Bowel Movement:

How many liquid bowel movements you had today?

| One: | Two: | Three: | Four: | More than 4: |

Did you have any of the followings today?

Bowel Urgency: YES NO
Bleeding: YES NO
Partial evacuation: YES NO
Sinking defecation: YES NO

Mucus in the stool: YES NO
Painful bowel movement: YES NO
High pressure evacuation: YES NO
Other Symptoms: YES NO

Stool Type:

1. Very constipated: YES NO
2. Constipated: YES NO
3. Normal sausage-like: YES NO
4. Normal smooth: YES NO
5. Soft blobs: YES NO
6. Mushy: YES NO
7. Liquid: YES NO
Any Notes:

Activities:

Did you have a workout today? YES NO
Was it intense? YES NO
How long did you have workout? ____ Min.
Your weight changed today? YES NO
Did you have a good appetite? YES NO
How many glasses of water did you have? _____
Did you have time to meditate or practice Yoga today? YES NO

Date: _____   Mon Tue Wed Thu Fri Sat Sun

Quote of the Day:

> "Stay close to anything that makes you glad you are alive."
> - Hafez

Your Mood Today

Stress Level: 0–10 (No Stress — Full Stress)

Sleep Quality: 0–10 (Very bad — Very well)

How long did you sleep last night? _____ Hrs.

Time	Meals Taken Today	Symptoms Experienced:	How intense? (1: low, 5: severe)
	Breakfast:		
	Lunch:		
	Dinner:		
	Snacks:		

Bowel Movement:

How many liquid bowel movements you had today?

| One: | Two: | Three: | Four: | More than 4: |

Did you have any of the followings today?

Bowel Urgency: YES NO
Bleeding: YES NO
Partial evacuation: YES NO
Sinking defecation: YES NO

Mucus in the stool: YES NO
Painful bowel movement: YES NO
High pressure evacuation: YES NO
Other Symptoms: YES NO

Stool Type:

1. Very constipated: YES NO
2. Constipated: YES NO
3. Normal sausage-like: YES NO
4. Normal smooth: YES NO
5. Soft blobs: YES NO
6. Mushy: YES NO
7. Liquid: YES NO
Any Notes:

Activities:

Did you have a workout today? YES NO
Was it intense? YES NO
How long did you have workout? _____ Min.
Your weight changed today? YES NO
Did you have a good appetite? YES NO
How many glasses of water did you have? _____
Did you have time to meditate or practice Yoga today? YES NO

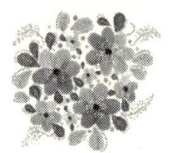

Week-12 IBS Control Record

Did you miss any activity due to your IBS condition?	YES NO
Do you think your IBS controlled well last week?	YES NO
Were you happy with your current treatment last week?	YES NO
Did you feel pain or discomfort last week?	YES NO
Did you have a good eating appetite last week?	YES NO
Did you feel fatigued last week?	YES NO
Did you feel depressed/anxious last week due to your IBS?	YES NO
Do you think you lost weight last week?	YES NO
Do you feel your bowel symptoms got better last week?	YES NO

Low FODMAP Diet Adherence:

Did you have any of the following foods this week?

Alcohol: YES NO	Chocolate: YES NO	Coffee: YES NO
Soda: YES NO	Sweet Fruits: YES NO	Lactose Products: YES NO
Fatty/greasy Foods: YES NO	Fried Foods: YES NO	Gluten Products: YES NO
FODMAP Sugars: YES NO	Raw Vegetables: YES NO	Spicy Foods: YES NO

Add any other suspicious foods you consumed: Did you get any discomfort?

1. _____ YES NO
2. _____ YES NO
3. _____ YES NO
4. _____ YES NO
5. _____ YES NO
6. _____ YES NO
7. _____ YES NO
8. _____ YES NO
9. _____ YES NO
10. _____ YES NO

Others:

Medications/Supplements taken this week: _____

Tell a good thing that happened this week: _____

Other Notes: _____

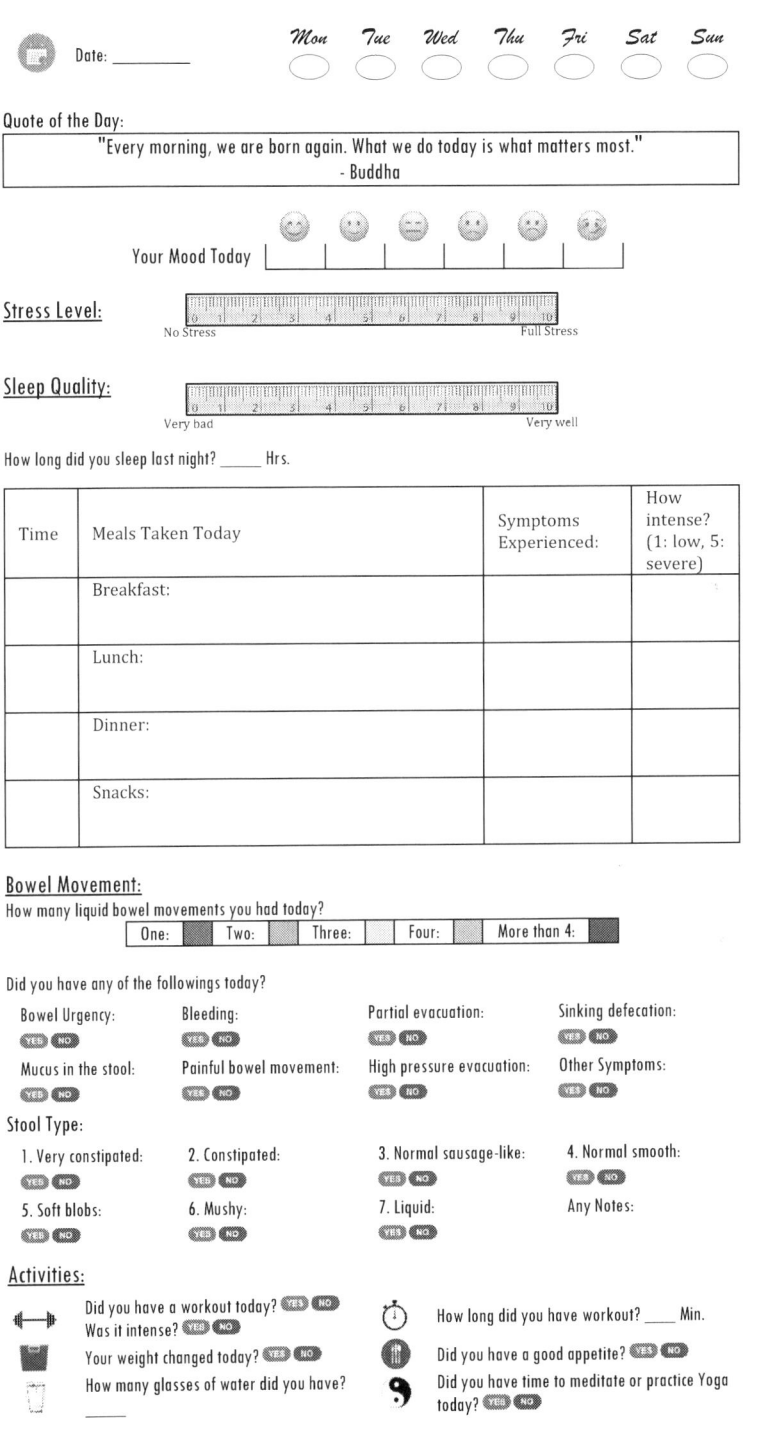

Date: _____   Mon Tue Wed Thu Fri Sat Sun

Quote of the Day:
> "Every morning, we are born again. What we do today is what matters most."
> - Buddha

Your Mood Today [ ] [ ] [ ] [ ] [ ] [ ]

Stress Level: 0 1 2 3 4 5 6 7 8 9 10
No Stress — Full Stress

Sleep Quality: 0 1 2 3 4 5 6 7 8 9 10
Very bad — Very well

How long did you sleep last night? _____ Hrs.

Time	Meals Taken Today	Symptoms Experienced:	How intense? (1: low, 5: severe)
	Breakfast:		
	Lunch:		
	Dinner:		
	Snacks:		

Bowel Movement:
How many liquid bowel movements you had today?
One: ___ Two: ___ Three: ___ Four: ___ More than 4: ___

Did you have any of the followings today?

Bowel Urgency: YES NO   Bleeding: YES NO   Partial evacuation: YES NO   Sinking defecation: YES NO
Mucus in the stool: YES NO   Painful bowel movement: YES NO   High pressure evacuation: YES NO   Other Symptoms: YES NO

Stool Type:

1. Very constipated: YES NO   2. Constipated: YES NO   3. Normal sausage-like: YES NO   4. Normal smooth: YES NO
5. Soft blobs: YES NO   6. Mushy: YES NO   7. Liquid: YES NO   Any Notes:

Activities:

Did you have a workout today? YES NO Was it intense? YES NO
Your weight changed today? YES NO
How many glasses of water did you have? _____

How long did you have workout? ____ Min.
Did you have a good appetite? YES NO
Did you have time to meditate or practice Yoga today? YES NO

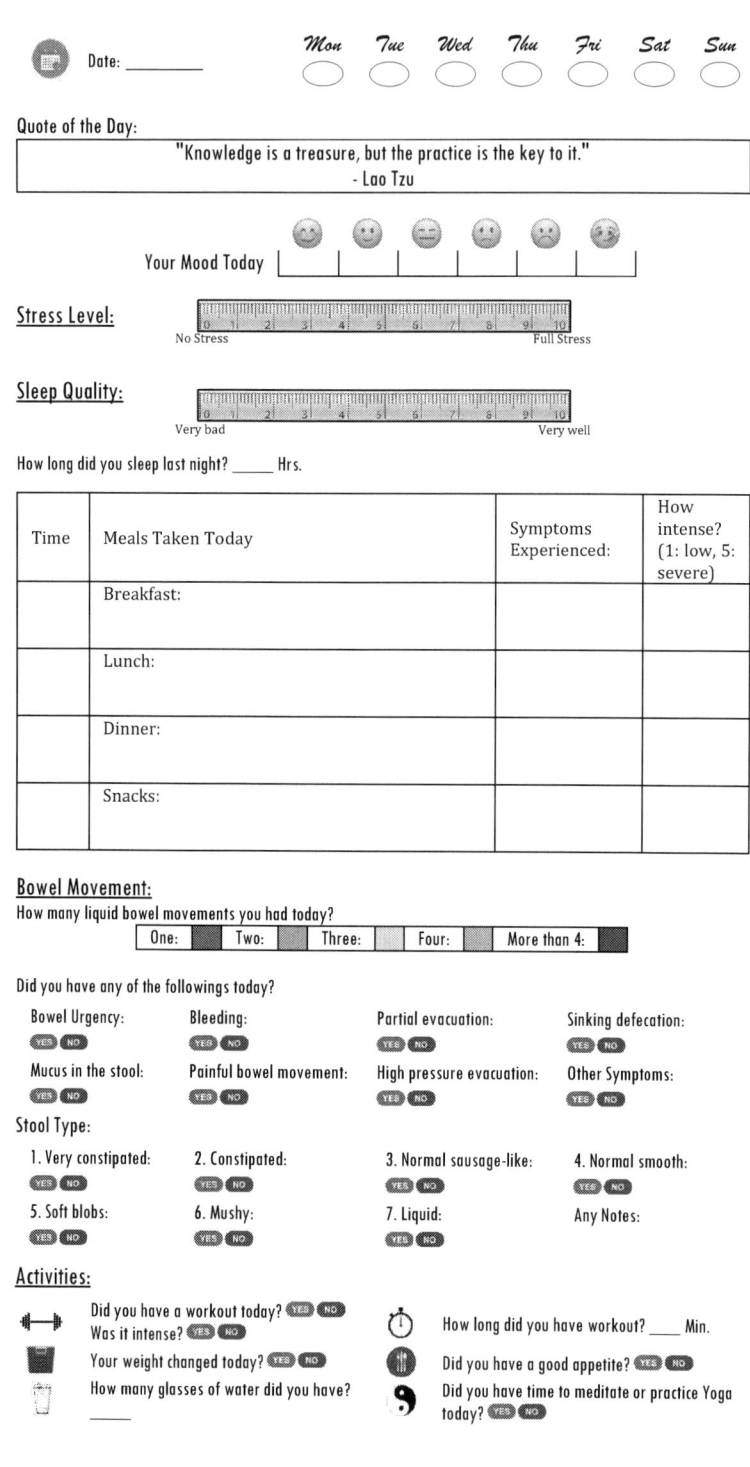

Date: _____   Mon Tue Wed Thu Fri Sat Sun

Quote of the Day:
"When the world pushes you to your knees, you're in the perfect position to pray."
- Rumi

Your Mood Today

Stress Level:
0 1 2 3 4 5 6 7 8 9 10
No Stress   Full Stress

Sleep Quality:
0 1 2 3 4 5 6 7 8 9 10
Very bad   Very well

How long did you sleep last night? _____ Hrs.

Time	Meals Taken Today	Symptoms Experienced:	How intense? (1: low, 5: severe)
	Breakfast:		
	Lunch:		
	Dinner:		
	Snacks:		

Bowel Movement:
How many liquid bowel movements you had today?

| One: | Two: | Three: | Four: | More than 4: |

Did you have any of the followings today?

Bowel Urgency: YES NO
Bleeding: YES NO
Partial evacuation: YES NO
Sinking defecation: YES NO

Mucus in the stool: YES NO
Painful bowel movement: YES NO
High pressure evacuation: YES NO
Other Symptoms: YES NO

Stool Type:

1. Very constipated: YES NO
2. Constipated: YES NO
3. Normal sausage-like: YES NO
4. Normal smooth: YES NO
5. Soft blobs: YES NO
6. Mushy: YES NO
7. Liquid: YES NO
Any Notes:

Activities:

Did you have a workout today? YES NO
Was it intense? YES NO
Your weight changed today? YES NO
How many glasses of water did you have? _____

How long did you have workout? _____ Min.
Did you have a good appetite? YES NO
Did you have time to meditate or practice Yoga today? YES NO

Date: _____   ○ Mon ○ Tue ○ Wed ○ Thu ○ Fri ○ Sat ○ Sun

Quote of the Day:

> "Thousands of candles can be lit from a single candle, and the life of the candle will not be shortened. Happiness never decreases by being shared." "Be vigilant; guard your mind against negative thoughts." - Buddha

Your Mood Today: [ ] [ ] [ ] [ ] [ ] [ ]

Stress Level: 0–10 (No Stress — Full Stress)

Sleep Quality: 0–10 (Very bad — Very well)

How long did you sleep last night? _____ Hrs.

Time	Meals Taken Today	Symptoms Experienced:	How intense? (1: low, 5: severe)
	Breakfast:		
	Lunch:		
	Dinner:		
	Snacks:		

Bowel Movement:

How many liquid bowel movements you had today?
One: ☐   Two: ☐   Three: ☐   Four: ☐   More than 4: ☐

Did you have any of the followings today?

Bowel Urgency: YES NO
Bleeding: YES NO
Partial evacuation: YES NO
Sinking defecation: YES NO

Mucus in the stool: YES NO
Painful bowel movement: YES NO
High pressure evacuation: YES NO
Other Symptoms: YES NO

Stool Type:

1. Very constipated: YES NO
2. Constipated: YES NO
3. Normal sausage-like: YES NO
4. Normal smooth: YES NO
5. Soft blobs: YES NO
6. Mushy: YES NO
7. Liquid: YES NO
Any Notes:

Activities:

Did you have a workout today? YES NO
Was it intense? YES NO
How long did you have workout? _____ Min.
Your weight changed today? YES NO
Did you have a good appetite? YES NO
How many glasses of water did you have? _____
Did you have time to meditate or practice Yoga today? YES NO

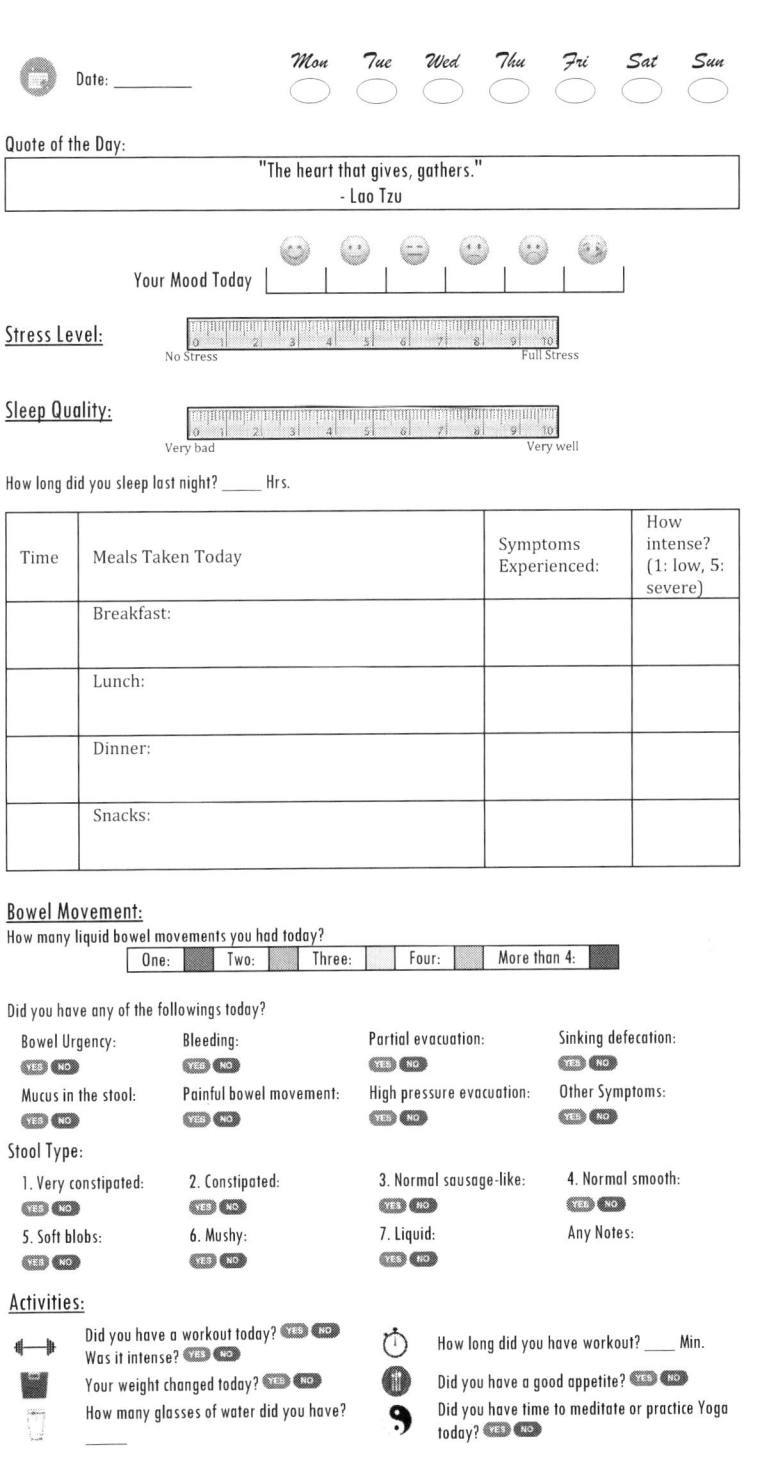

Date: _____   Mon Tue Wed Thu Fri Sat Sun

Quote of the Day:
"The heart that gives, gathers."
- Lao Tzu

Your Mood Today

Stress Level: 0 1 2 3 4 5 6 7 8 9 10
No Stress   Full Stress

Sleep Quality: 0 1 2 3 4 5 6 7 8 9 10
Very bad   Very well

How long did you sleep last night? _____ Hrs.

Time	Meals Taken Today	Symptoms Experienced:	How intense? (1: low, 5: severe)
	Breakfast:		
	Lunch:		
	Dinner:		
	Snacks:		

Bowel Movement:
How many liquid bowel movements you had today?
One: ___ Two: ___ Three: ___ Four: ___ More than 4: ___

Did you have any of the followings today?

Bowel Urgency: YES NO   Bleeding: YES NO   Partial evacuation: YES NO   Sinking defecation: YES NO
Mucus in the stool: YES NO   Painful bowel movement: YES NO   High pressure evacuation: YES NO   Other Symptoms: YES NO

Stool Type:
1. Very constipated: YES NO   2. Constipated: YES NO   3. Normal sausage-like: YES NO   4. Normal smooth: YES NO
5. Soft blobs: YES NO   6. Mushy: YES NO   7. Liquid: YES NO   Any Notes:

Activities:
Did you have a workout today? YES NO Was it intense? YES NO
How long did you have workout? _____ Min.
Your weight changed today? YES NO
Did you have a good appetite? YES NO
How many glasses of water did you have? _____
Did you have time to meditate or practice Yoga today? YES NO

Date: _____ ○ Mon ○ Tue ○ Wed ○ Thu ○ Fri ○ Sat ○ Sun

Quote of the Day:
"Don't move the way fear makes you move. Move the way love makes you move. Move the way joy makes you move." - Osho

Your Mood Today: 😊 🙂 😐 🙁 😣 😫

Stress Level: 0 1 2 3 4 5 6 7 8 9 10
No Stress — Full Stress

Sleep Quality: 0 1 2 3 4 5 6 7 8 9 10
Very bad — Very well

How long did you sleep last night? _____ Hrs.

Time	Meals Taken Today	Symptoms Experienced:	How intense? (1: low, 5: severe)
	Breakfast:		
	Lunch:		
	Dinner:		
	Snacks:		

Bowel Movement:

How many liquid bowel movements you had today?

| One: | Two: | Three: | Four: | More than 4: |

Did you have any of the followings today?

Bowel Urgency: YES NO
Bleeding: YES NO
Partial evacuation: YES NO
Sinking defecation: YES NO

Mucus in the stool: YES NO
Painful bowel movement: YES NO
High pressure evacuation: YES NO
Other Symptoms: YES NO

Stool Type:

1. Very constipated: YES NO
2. Constipated: YES NO
3. Normal sausage-like: YES NO
4. Normal smooth: YES NO
5. Soft blobs: YES NO
6. Mushy: YES NO
7. Liquid: YES NO
Any Notes:

Activities:

Did you have a workout today? YES NO
Was it intense? YES NO

How long did you have workout? _____ Min.

Your weight changed today? YES NO

Did you have a good appetite? YES NO

How many glasses of water did you have? _____

Did you have time to meditate or practice Yoga today? YES NO

Date: _____

Mon Tue Wed Thu Fri Sat Sun
 ○   ○   ○   ○   ○   ○   ○

Quote of the Day:
"Wherever you stand, be the soul of that place."
— Rumi

Your Mood Today | ☺ | ☺ | 😐 | ☹ | ☹ | 😄 |

Stress Level:
0 1 2 3 4 5 6 7 8 9 10
No Stress   Full Stress

Sleep Quality:
0 1 2 3 4 5 6 7 8 9 10
Very bad   Very well

How long did you sleep last night? _____ Hrs.

Time	Meals Taken Today	Symptoms Experienced:	How intense? (1: low, 5: severe)
	Breakfast:		
	Lunch:		
	Dinner:		
	Snacks:		

Bowel Movement:
How many liquid bowel movements you had today?
One: ▢ Two: ▢ Three: ▢ Four: ▢ More than 4: ▢

Did you have any of the followings today?

Bowel Urgency: YES NO
Bleeding: YES NO
Partial evacuation: YES NO
Sinking defecation: YES NO

Mucus in the stool: YES NO
Painful bowel movement: YES NO
High pressure evacuation: YES NO
Other Symptoms: YES NO

Stool Type:

1. Very constipated: YES NO
2. Constipated: YES NO
3. Normal sausage-like: YES NO
4. Normal smooth: YES NO
5. Soft blobs: YES NO
6. Mushy: YES NO
7. Liquid: YES NO
Any Notes:

Activities:

Did you have a workout today? YES NO
Was it intense? YES NO
Your weight changed today? YES NO
How many glasses of water did you have? _____

How long did you have workout? _____ Min.
Did you have a good appetite? YES NO
Did you have time to meditate or practice Yoga today? YES NO

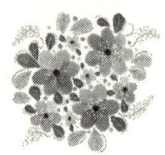

Week-13 IBS Control Record

Did you miss any activity due to your IBS condition?	YES NO
Do you think your IBS controlled well last week?	YES NO
Were you happy with your current treatment last week?	YES NO
Did you feel pain or discomfort last week?	YES NO
Did you have a good eating appetite last week?	YES NO
Did you feel fatigued last week?	YES NO
Did you feel depressed/anxious last week due to your IBS?	YES NO
Do you think you lost weight last week?	YES NO
Do you feel your bowel symptoms got better last week?	YES NO

Low FODMAP Diet Adherence:

Did you have any of the following foods this week?

Alcohol: YES NO	Chocolate: YES NO	Coffee: YES NO
Soda: YES NO	Sweet Fruits: YES NO	Lactose Products: YES NO
Fatty/greasy Foods: YES NO	Fried Foods: YES NO	Gluten Products: YES NO
FODMAP Sugars: YES NO	Raw Vegetables: YES NO	Spicy Foods: YES NO

Add any other suspicious foods you consumed: Did you get any discomfort?

1. _____ YES NO
2. _____ YES NO
3. _____ YES NO
4. _____ YES NO
5. _____ YES NO
6. _____ YES NO
7. _____ YES NO
8. _____ YES NO
9. _____ YES NO
10. _____ YES NO

Others:

Medications/Supplements taken this week: _____

Tell a good thing that happened this week: _____
_____

Other Notes: _____
_____
_____
_____
_____

Date: _____   Mon Tue Wed Thu Fri Sat Sun
                   ○   ○   ○   ○   ○   ○   ○

Quote of the Day:
> "An idea that is developed and put into action is more important than an idea that exists only as an idea." - Buddha

Your Mood Today | 😊 | 🙂 | 😐 | 🙁 | 😟 | 😫 |

Stress Level:
0 1 2 3 4 5 6 7 8 9 10
No Stress   Full Stress

Sleep Quality:
0 1 2 3 4 5 6 7 8 9 10
Very bad   Very well

How long did you sleep last night? _____ Hrs.

Time	Meals Taken Today	Symptoms Experienced:	How intense? (1: low, 5: severe)
	Breakfast:		
	Lunch:		
	Dinner:		
	Snacks:		

Bowel Movement:
How many liquid bowel movements you had today?
| One: | Two: | Three: | Four: | More than 4: |

Did you have any of the followings today?

Bowel Urgency: YES NO
Bleeding: YES NO
Partial evacuation: YES NO
Sinking defecation: YES NO

Mucus in the stool: YES NO
Painful bowel movement: YES NO
High pressure evacuation: YES NO
Other Symptoms: YES NO

Stool Type:

1. Very constipated: YES NO
2. Constipated: YES NO
3. Normal sausage-like: YES NO
4. Normal smooth: YES NO
5. Soft blobs: YES NO
6. Mushy: YES NO
7. Liquid: YES NO
Any Notes:

Activities:

Did you have a workout today? YES NO
Was it intense? YES NO
Your weight changed today? YES NO
How many glasses of water did you have? _____

How long did you have workout? ____ Min.
Did you have a good appetite? YES NO
Did you have time to meditate or practice Yoga today? YES NO

Date: _____   Mon Tue Wed Thu Fri Sat Sun
                 ○   ○   ○   ○   ○   ○   ○

Quote of the Day:
> "Never be ashamed of your tears... Be proud that you are still natural. Be proud that you can express the inexpressible through your tears." - Osho

Your Mood Today | 😊 | 🙂 | 😐 | 🙁 | 😣 |

Stress Level: 0 1 2 3 4 5 6 7 8 9 10
No Stress — Full Stress

Sleep Quality: 0 1 2 3 4 5 6 7 8 9 10
Very bad — Very well

How long did you sleep last night? _____ Hrs.

Time	Meals Taken Today	Symptoms Experienced:	How intense? (1: low, 5: severe)
	Breakfast:		
	Lunch:		
	Dinner:		
	Snacks:		

Bowel Movement:

How many liquid bowel movements you had today?

| One: | Two: | Three: | Four: | More than 4: |

Did you have any of the followings today?

Bowel Urgency: YES NO
Bleeding: YES NO
Partial evacuation: YES NO
Sinking defecation: YES NO

Mucus in the stool: YES NO
Painful bowel movement: YES NO
High pressure evacuation: YES NO
Other Symptoms: YES NO

Stool Type:

1. Very constipated: YES NO
2. Constipated: YES NO
3. Normal sausage-like: YES NO
4. Normal smooth: YES NO
5. Soft blobs: YES NO
6. Mushy: YES NO
7. Liquid: YES NO
Any Notes:

Activities:

Did you have a workout today? YES NO
Was it intense? YES NO
How long did you have workout? ____ Min.
Your weight changed today? YES NO
Did you have a good appetite? YES NO
How many glasses of water did you have? _____
Did you have time to meditate or practice Yoga today? YES NO

BIWEEKLY MEAL PLAN-1

Week-1:	*Week-2:*
Monday	**Monday**
Breakfast:	*Breakfast:*
Snack-1:	*Snack-1:*
Lunch:	*Lunch:*
Snack-2:	*Snack-2:*
Dinner:	*Dinner:*
Snack-3:	*Snack-3:*
Drinks:	*Drinks:*
Tuesday	**Tuesday**
Breakfast:	*Breakfast:*
Snack-1:	*Snack-1:*
Lunch:	*Lunch:*
Snack-2:	*Snack-2:*
Dinner:	*Dinner:*
Snack-3:	*Snack-3:*
Drinks:	*Drinks:*
Wednesday	**Wednesday**
Breakfast:	*Breakfast:*
Snack-1:	*Snack-1:*
Lunch:	*Lunch:*
Snack-2:	*Snack-2:*
Dinner:	*Dinner:*
Snack-3:	*Snack-3:*
Drinks:	*Drinks:*
Thursday	**Thursday**
Breakfast:	*Breakfast:*
Snack-1:	*Snack-1:*
Lunch:	*Lunch:*
Snack-2:	*Snack-2:*
Dinner:	*Dinner:*
Snack-3:	*Snack-3:*
Drinks:	*Drinks:*
Friday	**Friday**
Breakfast:	*Breakfast:*
Snack-1:	*Snack-1:*
Lunch:	*Lunch:*
Snack-2:	*Snack-2:*
Dinner:	*Dinner:*
Snack-3:	*Snack-3:*
Drinks:	*Drinks:*
Saturday	**Saturday**
Breakfast:	*Breakfast:*
Snack-1:	*Snack-1:*
Lunch:	*Lunch:*
Snack-2:	*Snack-2:*
Dinner:	*Dinner:*
Snack-3:	*Snack-3:*
Drinks:	*Drinks:*
Sunday	**Sunday**
Breakfast:	*Breakfast:*
Snack-1:	*Snack-1:*
Lunch:	*Lunch:*
Snack-2:	*Snack-2:*
Dinner:	*Dinner:*
Snack-3:	*Snack-3:*
Drinks:	*Drinks:*

BIWEEKLY MEAL PLAN-2

Week-1:	Week-2:
Monday	**Monday**
Breakfast:	Breakfast:
Snack-1:	Snack-1:
Lunch:	Lunch:
Snack-2:	Snack-2:
Dinner:	Dinner:
Snack-3:	Snack-3:
Drinks:	Drinks:
Tuesday	**Tuesday**
Breakfast:	Breakfast:
Snack-1:	Snack-1:
Lunch:	Lunch:
Snack-2:	Snack-2:
Dinner:	Dinner:
Snack-3:	Snack-3:
Drinks:	Drinks:
Wednesday	**Wednesday**
Breakfast:	Breakfast:
Snack-1:	Snack-1:
Lunch:	Lunch:
Snack-2:	Snack-2:
Dinner:	Dinner:
Snack-3:	Snack-3:
Drinks:	Drinks:
Thursday	**Thursday**
Breakfast:	Breakfast:
Snack-1:	Snack-1:
Lunch:	Lunch:
Snack-2:	Snack-2:
Dinner:	Dinner:
Snack-3:	Snack-3:
Drinks:	Drinks:
Friday	**Friday**
Breakfast:	Breakfast:
Snack-1:	Snack-1:
Lunch:	Lunch:
Snack-2:	Snack-2:
Dinner:	Dinner:
Snack-3:	Snack-3:
Drinks:	Drinks:
Saturday	**Saturday**
Breakfast:	Breakfast:
Snack-1:	Snack-1:
Lunch:	Lunch:
Snack-2:	Snack-2:
Dinner:	Dinner:
Snack-3:	Snack-3:
Drinks:	Drinks:
Sunday	**Sunday**
Breakfast:	Breakfast:
Snack-1:	Snack-1:
Lunch:	Lunch:
Snack-2:	Snack-2:
Dinner:	Dinner:
Snack-3:	Snack-3:
Drinks:	Drinks:

Low FODMAP Comprehensive Food List

High FODMAP Fruits (to avoid or to reduce)

Apples (all types)	Mango
Apricots	Nectarines
Avocado	Pawpaw (dried)
Bananas, ripe	Peaches
Blackberries	Pears
Blackcurrants	Persimmon
Boysenberry	Pineapple (dried)
Cherries	Plums
Currants	Pomegranate
Custard apple	Prunes
Dates	Raisins
Feijoa	Sea buckthorns
Figs	Sultanas
Goji berries	Tamarillo
Grapefruit	Tinned fruit in apple or pear juice
Guava (unripe)	Watermelon
Lychee	

**Fully avoid in any forms

Low FODMAP Fruits (to consume)

Ackee	Lemon & lemon juice
Bananas (unripe)	Lime & lime juice
Bilberries	Mandarin
Blueberries	Orange
Breadfruit	Passion fruit
Carambola	Pawpaw
Cantaloupe	Papaya
Cranberry (1 tbsp)	Pineapple
Clementine	Plantain (peeled)
Dragon fruit	Prickly pear
Lingonberries	Raspberry
Grapes	Rhubarb
Guava (ripe)	Strawberry
Honeydew melons	Tamarind
Kiwifruit	Tangelo

High FODMAP Vegetables and Legumes (to avoid or to reduce)

Vegetable		Vegetable	
Artichoke	R	Leek bulb	R
Asparagus	R	Mange Tout	R
Baked beans	R	Mixed vegetables	R
Beetroot (fresh)	R	Mung beans	R
Black eyed peas	R	Mushrooms	R
Broad beans	R	Onion (any forms)	R**
Butter beans	R	Peas, sugar snap	R
Cassava	R	Pickled vegetables	R
Cauliflower	R	Red kidney beans	R
Celery (> 5cm of stalk)	R	Savoy Cabbage	R
Choko	R	Soybeans or soya beans	R
Falafel	R	Split peas	R
Fermented cabbage (e.g. sauerkraut)	R	Scallions	R
Garlic (any forms, e.g., garlic powder)	R**	Spring Onions	R
Haricot beans	R	Shallots	R
Kidney beans	R	Taro	R
Lima beans	R		

**Fully avoid in any forms

Low FODMAP Vegetables and Legumes (to consume)

Vegetable		Vegetable	
Alfalfa	G	Lentils (small amounts)	G
Bamboo shoots	G	Lettuce (Normal)	G
Bean sprouts	G	Butter lettuce	G
Beetroot, canned, and/or pickled	G	Iceberg lettuce	G
Black beans (1/4 cup)	G	Radicchio lettuce	G
Bok choy	G	Red coral lettuce	G
Broccoli, whole (1/2 cup)	G	Rocket lettuce	G
Broccoli, heads (3/4 cup)	G	Romaine lettuce	G
Broccoli, stalks (1/2 cup)	G	Marrow	G
Broccolini, whole (1/2 cup), chopped	G	Okra	G
Broccolini, heads (1/2 cup)	G	Olives	G
Broccolini, stalks (1 cup)	G	Parsnip	G
Brussels sprouts (2 sprouts)	G	Peas, snow (5 pods)	G
Butternut squash (1/4 cup)	G	Pickled gherkins	G
Cabbage (up to 1 cup)	G	Pickled onions (large)	G
Callaloo	G	Potato	G
Carrots	G	Pumpkin	G
Celeriac	G	Pumpkin canned (1/4 cup)	G
Celery (< 5cm of stalk)	G	Radish	G
Chicory leaves	G	Red peppers, red bell pepper, & red capsicum	G

Chickpeas (1/4 cup)	G	Scallions, spring onions (green parts)	G
Chilli (if tolerable)	G	Seaweed, nori	G
Chives	G	Silverbeet, chard	G
Chocho (1/2 cup diced)	G	Spaghetti squash	G
Choy sum	G	Spinach, baby spinach	G
Collard greens	G	Squash	G
Corn / sweet corn – if tolerable & only in small amounts (e.g., 1/2 cob)	G	Sundried tomatoes (4 pieces)	G
Courgette	G	Swede	G
Eggplant	G	Swiss chard	G
Fennel	G	Sweet potato (1/2 cup)	G
Green beans	G	Tomato (canned, cherry, common, & roma)	G
Green pepper, green bell pepper, green capsicum	G	Tomatillos (canned)	G
Ginger	G	Turnip	G
Kale	G	Water chestnuts	G
Karela	G	Yam	G
Leek leaves	G	Zucchini	G

Fish, Seafood, Meats and Poultry to Consume and to Avoid

Beef	G	Canned tuna	G
Chicken	G	Fresh fish	G
Chorizo		• Cod	G
Cold Cuts	G	• Haddock	G
Deli Meats	G	• Plaice	G
Foie gras	G	• Salmon	G
Ham Cuts	G	• Trout	G
Kangaroo	G	• Tuna	G
Lamb	G	Seafood (make sure nothing else is added)	G
Pork	G	• Crab	G
Prosciutto	G	• Lobster	G
Quorn, mince	G	• Mussels	G
Sausage		• Oysters	G
Turkey, Turkey Cuts	G	• Prawns	G
Processed meat (always check ingredients)	G	• Shrimp	G

Dairy Foods and Eggs (to eat and to avoid)

Buttermilk		Butter		• Almond milk
Cheese, cream		Cheese:		• Hemp milk
Cheese, Halmoumi		• Brie		• Lactose free milk
Cheese, ricotta		• Camembert		• Macadamia milk
Cream		• Cheddar		• Oat milk (30 ml)
Custard		• Cottage (2 tbs)		• Rice milk (up to 200ml)
Gelato		• Feta		Sorbet
Ice cream		• Goat or chevre		Soy protein (not soya beans)
Kefir		• Monterey Jack		Swiss cheese
Milk:		• Mozzarella		Tempeh
Cow milk		• Parmesan		Tofu (drained and firm varieties)
Goat milk		• Ricotta (2 tbs)		Whipped cream
Evaporated milk		• Swiss		Coconut yogurt
Sheep's milk		Dairy free chocolate pudding		• Greek yogurt (small amounts)
Sour cream		Eggs		• Lactose-free yogurt
Yoghurt		Margarine		• Goats yogurt

Grains, Breads, Cookies, Nuts, Pastas, and Cakes (to avoid or to reduce)

Wheat Products:		Bread:	
• Biscuits or cookies including chocolate chip cookies		• Granary bread	
• Bread, wheat (>1 slice)		• Multigrain bread	
• Breadcrumbs		• Naan	
• Cakes		• Oatmeal bread	
• Cereal bar (wheat-based)		• Pumpernickel bread	
• Croissants		• Roti	
• Crumpets		• Sourdough with Kamut	
Egg noodles		Cashews	
Muffins		Chestnut flour	
Pastries		Couscous	
Pasta, wheat (>0.5 cup cooked)		Einkorn flour	
Udon noodles		Freekeh	
• Wheat bran		Gnocchi	
• Wheat cereals		Granola bar	
• Wheat flour		Muesli cereal	
• Wheat germ		Muesli bar	
• Wheat noodles		Pistachios	

• Wheat rolls	Rye	
Almond meal	Rye crispbread	
Amaranth flour	Semolina	
Barley including flour	Spelt flour	
Bran cereals		

Grains, Breads, Cookies, Nuts, Pastas, and Cakes (to consume)

Wheat free breads	Oats	
• Gluten free breads	Oatcakes	
• Bread:	Peanuts	
• Corn bread	Pecans (maximum of 15)	
• Oat bread	Pine nuts (maximum of 15)	
• Rice bread	Polenta	
• Spelt sourdough bread	Popcorn	
• Potato flour bread	Porridge & oat-based cereals	
Wheat free or gluten free pasta	Potato flour	
Bread, wheat (1 slice)	Pretzels	
Almonds (maximum 15)	Quinoa	
Biscuit, savoury	Pasta, wheat (>1/2 cup cooked)	
Biscuit, shortbread (only 1)	Rice:	
Brazil nuts	• Basmati rice	
Bulgur (1/4 cup cooked)	• Brown rice	
Buckwheat	• Rice noodles	
Buckwheat flour	• White rice	
Buckwheat noodles	• Rice bran	
Brown rice or whole grain rice	• Rice cakes	
Chestnuts	• Rice crackers	
Chips, plain potato crisps	• Rice flakes	
Cornflour	• Rice flour	
Crispbread	• Rice Krispies	
Corncakes	Seeds:	
Cornflakes (1/2 cup)	• Chia seeds	
Cornflakes, gluten free	• Egusi seeds	
Coconut milk, cream, flesh	• Hemp seeds	
Corn, creamed and canned (> 1/3 cup)	• Poppy seeds	
Corn tortillas (3 tortillas)	• Pumpkin seeds	
Crackers, plain	• Sesame seeds	
Flax seeds (>1 tbsp)	• Sunflower seeds	
Hazelnuts (maximum of 15)	Starch, maize, potato & tapioca	
Macadamia nuts	Sorghum	
Millet	Tortilla chips & corn chips	
Mixed nuts	Walnuts	
Oatmeal (1/2 cup)		

Dips, Sweeteners, Sweets, and Spreads (to avoid or to reduce)

Agave	Relish or vegetable pickle
Caviar dip	Stock cubes
Fructose	Sugar-free sweets containing polyols ending in -ol or isomalt
Fruit bar	Sweeteners with E numbers:
Gravy, if it contains onion	• Inulin
High fructose corn syrup (HFCS)	• Isomalt (E953/953)
Hummus	• Lactitol (E966/966)
Honey	• Maltitol (E965/965)
Jam, mixed berries	• Mannitol (E241/421)
Jam, strawberry with HFCS	• Sorbitol (E420/420)
Molasses	• Xylitol (E967/967)
Pesto sauce	Tahini paste
Quince paste	Tzatziki dip

Dips, Sweeteners, Sweets, and Spreads (to consume)

Aspartame	Miso paste
Acesulfame K	Mustard
Almond butter	Oyster sauce
Barbecue sauce (check label)	Pesto sauce (>1 tbsp)
Capers (in vinegar)	Peanut butter
Capers (salted)	Rice malt syrup
Chocolate:	Saccharine
• Dark chocolate	Shrimp paste
• Milk chocolate (3 squares)	Soy sauce
• White chocolate (3 squares)	Sriracha hot chilli sauce (1 tsp)
Chutney (1 tablespoon)	Stevia
Dijon mustard	Sweet & sour sauce
Erythritol (E968/968)	Sucralose
Fish sauce	Sugar (white)
Golden syrup	Tamarind paste
Glucose	Tomato sauce (2 sachets)
Glycerol (E422/422)	Vegemite
Jam or jelly (strawberry)	Vinegars:
Ketchup (1 sachet)	• Apple cider vinegar (2 tbsp)
Maple syrup	• Balsamic vinegar (2 tbsp)
Marmalade	• Rice wine vinegar
Marmite	Wasabi
Mayonnaise – make sure no garlic or onion in ingredients	Worcestershire sauce

Drinks, and Protein Powders (to eat and to avoid)

Avoid		Eat	
Beer (more than one bottle)		Alcohol is an irritant to the gut (limit the intake)	G
Coconut water		Beer (limit it to one drink)	G
Cordial, apple and raspberry (with 50-100% real juice)		Vodka (or clear spirits)	G
Cordial, orange (with 25-50% real juice)		Gin	G
Fruit & herbal teas with apple		Whiskey	G
Fruit juices (large quantities)		Wine (limit it to one drink)	G
Fruit juices with apple, pear, or mango		Water	R
Kombucha		Espresso coffee (regular or decaffeinated, black)	G
Malted chocolate flavored drink		Espresso coffee (with up to 250ml lactose-free milk)	G
Meal replacement drinks with milk-based products (e.g. Ensure, Slim Fast)		Instant coffee (regular or decaffeinated, black)	G
Orange juice (>100ml)		Instant coffee (with up to 250ml lactose-free milk)	G
Quinoa milk		Drinking chocolate powder	G
Rum		Fruit juice (125ml only safe fruits)	G
Sodas cwith High Fructose Corn Syrup (HFCS)		Kvass	G
Soymilk with soy beans		Lemonade (low quantities)	G
Sports drinks		Protein powders:	
Whey protein (hydrolyzed unless lactose-free)		• Egg protein	G
• Black tea with added soymilk		• Pea protein (up to 20g)	G
• Chai tea (strong)		• Rice protein	G
• Dandelion tea (strong)		• Sacha Inchi protein	G
• Fennel tea		• Whey protein isolate	G
• Chamomile tea		Soya milk made with soy protein	G
• Herbal tea (strong)		Sugar free fizzy drinks, soft drinks, soda: e.g., diet coke, (only low quantities)	G
• Oolong Tea		Sugar fizzy drinks, soft drinks, soda with no HFCS: e.g., lemonade, & cola. Limit intake as they are unhealthy and gut irritant	G
Wine (> one glass)		Tea: white, green, peppermint, & chai tea (weak)	G
Whey protein (concentrate unless lactose-free)		Black tea (weak e.g., PG Tips)	G

Prebiotics, Cooking ingredients, Herbs and Spices (to eat and to avoid)

Acai powder	G
Asafoetida powder (an ecellent onion substitute)	G
Baking powder	G
Baking soda	G
Cacao powder	G
Carob Powder	
Cocoa powder	G
Cream, 2 tablespoons	G
FOS – fructooligosaccharides (in prebiotics)	
Gelatine	G
Ghee	G
Icing sugar	G
Inulin in prebiotics	
Lard	G
Nutritional yeast	G
Oligofructose (in Prebiotics)	
Salt	G
Soybean oil	G
Oils: Avocado oil, Canola oil, Coconut oil, Olive oil, Peanut oil, Rice bran oil, Sesame oil, Soybean oil, Sunflower oil, & Vegetable oil	G
Spices: All spice, Black pepper, Cardamon, Chilli powder (check ingredients, sometimes has garlic added), Cinnamon, Cloves, Cumin, Curry powder, Fennel seeds, Five spice, Goraka, Mustard seeds, Nutmeg, Paprika, Saffron, Star anise, & Turmeric	G
Herbs: Basil, Bay leaves, Cilantro, Coriander, Curry leaves, Fenugreek, Gotukala, Lemongrass, Mint, Oregano, Pandan, Parsley, Rampa, Rosemary, Sage, Tarragon, & Thyme	G

Notes...

Notes...

Last Words...

The author of this journal would like to thank you for purchasing and reading this journal and hope the journal was helpful to you. If you found this journal useful or learned something from it, It would be much appreciated if you write a short review on the Amazon website.

The success of such medical journals highly depends on your honest reviews. Your reviews can help the author improve the quality of this journal in the next revisions. It can also help other people to make informed decisions about having this journal as well. If you have any feedback, comments or questions, feel free to email Monet Manbacci: monetmanbacci@gmail.com

Thanks again for your support!

About The Author

Monet Manbacci, Ph.D., is the author of *Crohn's Disease Comprehensive Diet Guide and CookBook*, *The Comprehensive Guide to Crohn's Disease*, *Ulcerative Colitis Comprehensive Diet Guide and Cookbook*, and *My IBS Management Journal* Books. He has a Doctor of Philosophy (Ph.D.) degree in Applied Sciences and has been involved in academic and scientific research for more than 14 years. He is one of the IBD patients that initially had been diagnosed with IBS.

Other Books By Monet Manbacci

The Comprehensive Guide to Crohn's Disease, All You Need to Know About Crohn's Disease, from Diagnosis to Management & Treatment (Autoimmune Disease Series Book 1), by Monet Manbacci, P.h.D., Amazon Publishing, 2019.

Crohn's Disease Comprehensive Diet Guide and Cook Book: More Than130 Recipes and 75 Essential Cooking Tips For Crohn's Patients (Autoimmune Disease Series Book 2), by Monet Manbacci, P.h.D., Amazon Publishing, 2019.

Ulcerative Colitis Comprehensive Diet Guide and Cook Book (Autoimmune Disease Series Book 3), by Monet Manbacci, P.h.D., Amazon Publishing, 2019

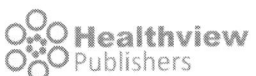

Manufactured by Amazon.ca
Bolton, ON